Revision Clinical Ophthalmology

Daniel B. Byles MA FRCOphth
Eye Hospital, Radcliffe Infirmary, Oxford, UK

S. James Talks MA MRCP FRCOphth
Eye Hospital, Radcliffe Infirmary, Oxford, UK

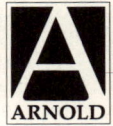

A member of the Hodder Headline Group
LONDON • SYDNEY • AUCKLAND
Co-published in the USA by Oxford University Press, Inc., New York

Dedicated to Megan and Kate

First published in Great Britain in 1998 by
Arnold, a division of Hodder Headline PLC,
338 Euston Road, London NW1 3BH
http://www.arnoldpublishers.com

Co-published in the United States of America by
Oxford University Press Inc.,
198 Madison Avenue, New York, NY 10016

© 1998 Daniel B. Byles and S. James Talks

All rights reserved. No part of this publication may be reproduced or transmitted in any form or by any means, electronically or mechanically, including photocopying, recording or any information storage or retrieval system, without either prior permission in writing from the publisher or a licence permitting restricted copying. In the United Kingdom such licences are issued by the Copyright Licensing Agency: 90 Tottenham Court Road, London W1P 9HE.

While the advice and information in this book is believed to be true and accurate at the date of going to press, neither the authors nor the publisher can accept any legal responsibility or liability for any errors or omissions that may be made. In particular (but without limiting the generality of the preceding disclaimer) every effort has been made to check drug dosages; however it is still possible that errors have been missed. Furthermore, dosage schedules are constantly being revised and new side-effects recognized. For these reasons the reader is strongly urged to consult the drug companies' printed instructions before administering any of the drugs recommended in this book.

British Library Cataloguing in Publication Data
A catalogue entry for this book is available from the British Library

Library of Congress Cataloging-in-Publication Data
A catalog record for this book is available from the Library of Congress

ISBN 0 340 70577 9

1 2 3 4 5   95 96 97 98 99

Publisher: Georgina Bentliff
Production Editor: James Rabson
Production Controller: Helen Whitehorn
Cover designer: Terry Griffiths

Typeset in 10/12 pt Helvetica by Prepress Projects, Perth, Scotland
Printed and bound in the United Kingdom by JW Arrowsmith Ltd, Bristol

Contents

Preface	iv
Acknowledgements	v
Questions grouped by topic	vi
Paper 1	1
Paper 2	15
Paper 3	29
Answers to Paper 1	42
Answers to Paper 2	64
Answers to Paper 3	86

Preface

This book aims to provide clearly thought out, up-to-date and practical ophthalmic information in multiple-choice format. Multiple choice forms a major part of the Fellowship examinations and requires a good factual knowledge as well as familiarity with this type of examination. This book provides the opportunity to practise papers and also contains information that will be useful for the vivas and clinical examinations.

The book contains three papers of 60 questions with the answers at the end. Each question has five stems that may each be answered true or false. Remember that the Fellowship examination papers are negatively marked, with a mark deducted from your score for each incorrect response. For this reason you should only answer a stem if you are sure of the correct answer or are confident of your 'guess'. There is no absolute pass mark for the examination but you should aim to get at least two or three positive marks for each question. When using this book you can either practise doing individual papers, or, if you wish to revise a particular topic separately, a list of question numbers under different subject headings is given at the beginning. Although by no means comprehensive, this book covers a wide range of relevant topics and may highlight areas where more reading is required. It also contains information from recent literature and published guidelines that is often not readily available in standard textbooks.

Daniel B. Byles and S. James Talks
June 1998

ACKNOWLEDGEMENTS

We would like to acknowledge Mr J. F. Salmon, MD FRCS FRCOphth and Mr J. S. Elston BSc MD FRCS FRCOphth, Consultant Ophthalmologists at the Oxford Eye Hospital, for their help in the preparation of this book.

Questions Grouped by Topic

Topic	Question numbers
Eyelids/lacrimal	1, 2, 3, 61, 62, 121, 122
Orbital	4, 5, 6, 63, 64, 65, 123, 124, 125, 162
Conjunctiva, cornea and sclera	7, 8, 9, 10, 11, 12, 66, 67, 68, 69, 70, 71, 72, 73, 126, 127, 128, 129, 130, 131, 132, 158, 179
Lens/cataract	13, 14, 74, 75, 133
Glaucoma	15, 16, 17, 18, 76, 77, 78, 79, 134, 135, 136, 137, 138
Uvea	19, 20, 21, 22, 28, 60, 80, 81, 82, 83, 139, 140, 141, 151
Medical retina	14, 23, 24, 25, 26, 27, 28, 29, 30, 31, 32, 83, 84, 85, 86, 87, 88, 89, 90, 91, 92, 93, 142, 143, 144, 145, 146, 147, 148, 149, 152
Vitreo-retinal	33, 34, 35, 94, 95, 96, 153, 154, 155
Strabismus	36, 37, 38, 97, 98, 99, 100, 107, 156, 157
Paediatric	39, 40, 41, 75, 93, 100, 101, 102, 103, 156, 159, 160, 161, 162, 173
Neuro-ophthalmology and systemic	42, 43, 44, 45, 46, 47, 48, 49, 50, 51, 52, 53, 104, 105, 106, 107, 108, 109, 110, 111, 112, 113, 114, 115, 116, 163, 164, 165, 166, 167, 168, 169, 170, 171, 172, 173
General	54, 55, 56, 57, 117, 118, 150, 158, 174, 175, 176, 177, 178
Pathology	2, 58, 59, 60, 119, 120, 179, 180

PAPER 1

Questions

1 Regarding eyelid lesions,

    A keratoacanthomas enlarge more slowly than squamous cell carcinomas
    B squamous cell carcinomas are the most common form of malignant lesion
    C molluscum contagiosum often causes a follicular conjunctivitis
    D a basal cell carcinoma near the medial canthus is more likely to invade the orbit than one situated elsewhere
    E sebaceous cell carcinoma should be suspected in recurrent chalazion

2 Basal cell carcinomas of the eyelid

    A are commonest on the upper lid
    B are commonly found in patients with xeroderma pigmentosum
    C of the morpheiform type show marked peripheral pallisading on histology
    D recur least frequently after surgical excision
    E may have excessive removal of healthy tissue when treated with Mohs' micrographic surgery

3 Causes of acquired canalicular obstruction include:

    A pemphigoid
    B rheumatoid arthritis
    C herpes simplex
    D topical steroid drops
    E lacrimal syringing

4 The following features of proptosis are consistent with the diagnoses given:

    A unilateral presentation and thyroid eye disease
    B axial proptosis and a sinus mucocele
    C pulsatile proptosis and neurofibromatosis
    D a bruit and a carotico-cavernous fistula
    E associated sinus and chest lesions and Wegener's granulomatosis

5   In cases when removal of an eye is required,

   A   enucleation is preferable to evisceration in severely traumatized eyes
   B   an adult-sized implant should be placed as early as possible in a young child
   C   evisceration is suitable for ciliary body melanoma
   D   hydroxyapatite implants have a slightly higher rate of early exposure than ball implants
   E   evisceration is preferable to enucleation in cases of endophthalmitis

6   Comparing orbital with preseptal cellulitis,

   A   both originate most commonly from sinus infections
   B   ocular movements are normal in preseptal cellulitis
   C   the globe is usually involved in preseptal cellulitis
   D   vision is more likely to be reduced in orbital cellulitis
   E   the eyelids are unaffected in orbital cellulitis

7   In astigmatic keratotomy

   A   keratoconus may be treated in its early stages
   B   elderly patients are more liable to overcorrection
   C   the incision should not exceed 70% of corneal thickness
   D   '1:1 coupling' means that for each dioptre of astigmatism corrected the spherical equivalent changes by 1 dioptre
   E   incisions should not cross other corneal incisions

8   With regard to corneal grafting,

   A   corneal graft rejection is largely T cell mediated
   B   only class 2 MHCs are expressed in the corneal stroma
   C   tissue typing is routinely performed for high-risk grafts
   D   early graft failure (within 10 days) is usually because of rejection
   E   more than 50% of graft rejection occurs within the first 6 months

9   Regarding corneal dystrophies,

   A   macular dystrophy presents late in life
   B   granular dystrophy often causes severe visual impairment

C lattice dystrophy is liable to recur in a graft
D Schnyder's crystalline dystrophy is associated with hypercholesterolaemia
E Reis–Buckler's dystrophy is autosomal recessive

10   Causes of dry eye include:

A graft versus host disease
B sarcoidosis
C ocular chemical burn
D Wegener's granulomatosis
E calcium channel-blocking drugs

11   Regarding ocular surface disorders,

A sodium versenate (EDTA) is an effective treatment for Salzman's nodular degeneration
B patching is a cause of filamentary keratitis
C primary amyloid can be deposited in the conjunctiva
D the local application of mitomycin C can be used to prevent pterygium recurrence
E band-shaped keratopathy may be removed by excimer laser

12   *Acanthamoeba* keratitis

A is slowly progressive and not painful
B is always associated with contact lenses
C may cause scleritis
D can cause corneal perineural infiltrates
E can be diagnosed on corneal biopsy and staining with calcofluor white

13   In a patient with subluxated lenses,

A a positive urine sodium nitroprusside test suggests Weill–Marchesani syndrome
✓B accommodation is usually retained in Marfan's syndrome
C with homocystinuria, the displacement is usually superior
✓D Marfan's syndrome is the commonest cause in childhood
✓E with homocystinuria, pyridoxine (vitamin B6) therapy may delay mental retardation

14 Regarding cystoid macular oedema (CMO) following cataract surgery,

   A the incidence is higher with primary posterior capsulotomy or vitreous loss
   B the peak incidence is 2 weeks post-operatively
   C angiographic CMO is less common than clinical CMO
   D older patients are at increased risk
   E lamellar holes develop in 70% of cases

15 In managing a case of low-tension glaucoma, in which there is progression of visual field loss, the following should be considered:

   A measuring the 24-hour ambulatory blood pressure
   B asking if the patient suffers from migraine
   C phasing
   D aiming to control the intra-ocular pressure at 18 mmHg
   E asking if the patient is using nasal steroid sprays

16 With glaucomatous optic nerve damage,

   A fibres from the papillomacular bundle are the most sensitive to glaucomatous damage
   B peripapillary atrophy is significantly associated with field loss in low-tension glaucoma
   C notching of the disc occurs most commonly nasally
   D optic disc cupping is reversible in some cases
   E disc changes can be detected before field changes

17 With the pseudoexfoliation syndrome,

   A exfoliative material can be found in subconjunctival tissue
   B iris transillumination occurs especially in the periphery
   C phacodonesis can occur
   D lens extraction can help the condition
   E patients are usually elderly at presentation

18 The following mechanisms of glaucoma are correctly associated:

   A rubeosis iridis causes angle-closure glaucoma
   B phacomorphic glaucoma is a form of acute secondary angle-closure glaucoma

C the Posner–Schlossman syndrome is associated with intermittent angle closure
D uveitis can cause angle-closure glaucoma without pupil block
E if a carotico-cavernous fistula causes glaucoma it is usually open-angle glaucoma

19 The following factors are associated with a poor prognosis in choroidal malignant melanoma:

A rapid tumour regression after radiotherapy
B advanced patient age at enucleation
C lymphocytic infiltration of tumour
D increased number of epithelioid cells per high-power field
E the presence of closed vascular loops

20 The following statements about choroidal naevi are true:

A 10% of all naevi progress to malignant melanomas
B B-scan ultrasonography is a useful test in the routine assessment of naevi
C the presence of lipofuscin suggests the possibility of malignant progression
D choroidal naevi may be present in 2% of the population
E the presence of surface drusen is a worrying feature

21 The following tests may be appropriate in a patient with uveitis:

A angiotensin-converting enzyme (ACE) level for suspected Behçet's syndrome
B *Toxoplasma* serology
C VDRL (Venereal Disease Research Laboratory) for anterior uveitis
D HLA B27 in Reiter's syndrome
E serum calcium for sarcoidosis

22 Regarding pars planitis,

A it is usually unilateral
B cystoid macular oedema is an important cause of visual loss
C peripheral venous sheathing may occur
D sarcoidosis is a possible differential diagnosis
E it typically starts in middle age

23 Typical causes of visual loss after branch retinal vein occlusion include:

   A macular oedema
   B neovascular glaucoma
   C vitreous haemorrhage
   D foveal ischaemia
   E lipid exudation

24 The following signs may be caused by systemic hypertension:

   A cottonwool spots
   B macular star
   C bull's-eye maculopathy
   D Elschnig's spots
   E optic disc swelling

25 Indications for laser treatment of macular oedema according to the Early Treatment for Diabetic Retinopathy Study (ETDRS) include:

   A enlargement of the foveal avascular zone on fluorescein angiography
   B retinal thickening (oedema) within 500 µm of the centre of the fovea
   C retinal thickening of one disc diameter or larger within the temporal arcades
   D hard exudate within 500 µm of the centre of the fovea if associated with adjacent retinal thickening (oedema)
   E microaneurysms within 500 µm of the centre of the fovea

26 The following factors relate to the prognosis of diabetic retinopathy:

   A intraretinal microvascular abnormalities (IRMAs) are a poor prognostic sign in non-proliferative retinopathy
   B improvement in blood sugar control reduces the onset and progression of diabetic retinopathy
   C rapid improvement in blood sugar control may worsen retinopathy
   D control of hypertension may reduce the progression of retinopathy in the long term
   E proteinuria is a poor prognostic sign

Paper 1 *Questions*

27   Causes of visual loss associated with sickle cell (SC) disease include:

   A   rhegmatogenous retinal detachment
   B   subretinal neovascularization
   C   ischaemic optic neuropathy
   D   macular branch artery occlusion
   E   vitreous haemorrhage

28   Regarding punctate inner choroidopathy (PIC),

   ✓A   it is associated with choroidal neovascularization
   B   it is associated with an active vitritis
   C   it is more common in older hypermetropic men
   D   it is due to histoplasmosis
   E   enlargement of the blind spot is a recognized feature

29   Causes of a retinitis pigmentosa-like pigmentation include:

   ✓A   spontaneous retinal reattachment
   ✓B   syphilis
   ✓C   quinine
   D   Niemann–Pick disease
   E   Fabry's disease

30   With a central retinal vein occlusion (CRVO),

   A   macular grid laser is recommended for persistent macular oedema
   ✓B   pan-retinal photocoagulation may be effective treatment for iris neovascularization
   ✓C   the risk of neovascular glaucoma is about 50% in ischaemic CRVO
   D   a hemicentral retinal vein occlusion has similar aetiological risk factors to a branch vein occlusion
   E   retinal new vessels usually arise before anterior segment new vessels

✓31   Retinal vascular occlusions

   ✓A   may occur with activated protein C resistance
   B   with a history of recurrent spontaneous abortions suggest a diagnosis of antithrombin III deficiency

C occur with increased frequency in Christmas disease (haemophilia B)
D occur with increased frequency in sickle cell disease ✓
E may occur with the antiphospholipid syndrome ✓

32 The following statements about Best's vitelliform macular dystrophy are true:

A the electro-oculogram (EOG) is normal in the early stages
B 50% of siblings of a patient will have inherited the risk of developing Best's disease
C the lesions may be multiple
D there is a risk of choroidal neovascularization
E nystagmus is a typical feature

33 With regard to ocular perforation and intra-ocular foreign bodies (IOFBs),

A plain frontal and lateral X-rays should be performed where an IOFB is suspected
B removal via pars plana magnet extraction is indicated for IOFBs embedded in the retina at the posterior pole
C shallowing of the anterior chamber is usually seen in posterior segment perforation
D magnetic resonance imaging (MRI) is the best technique for accurately localizing the IOFB
E *Bacillus cereus* is a common cause of post-perforation endophthalmitis

34 The following statements about proliferative vitreoretinopathy (PVR) are true:

A longstanding retinal detachments (RDs) are at lower risk
B rigidity of the detached retina is a feature ✓
C 1% of retinal detachments develop PVR
D large retinal breaks are often present ✓
E retinal star folds are the earliest sign

35 Causes of exudative retinal detachments include:

A pre-eclampsia ✓
B hypoproteinaemia ✓
C hyperthyroidism
D scleritis ✓
E Vogt–Koyanagi–Harada syndrome ✓

36 In the assessment of strabismus,

   A the presence of dissociated vertical deviation (DVD) suggests that an esotropia is congenital
   B to measure an esotropia with a prism cover test the prism should be held base-in in front of the deviating eye
   C the larger pattern plotted on a Hess chart is of the eye with the paretic muscle
   D a pen torch is a good target for a cover test looking for an accommodative esotropia
   E a child with a congenital esotropia may appear to be unable to abduct

37 Microtropia

   A is usually diagnosed with a cover test using a 20-dioptre prism
   B is usually associated with anisometropia
   C often requires surgery
   D is associated with DVD
   E is usually an exotropia

38 A chin-down head posture may be due to

   A an A exotropia
   B an A esotropia
   C bilateral IV nerve palsies
   D down-beat nystagmus
   E an internuclear ophthalmoplegia

39 Regarding delayed visual maturation,

   A it may be associated with ocular disease
   B it has a worse prognosis when it is an isolated finding
   C it may lead to subnormal vision in adulthood
   D when associated with mental disease the visual performance may be improved by repeating the test in a noisy environment
   E electrophysiological testing may show persistence of juvenile waveforms on visual evoked potential (VEP)

40 In the congenital rubella syndrome,

   A infection later in pregnancy results in more severe ocular complications
   B virus may be cultured from lens aspirate at 4 years of age
   C pigmentary retinopathy is the most common ocular finding
   D when pigment mottling is present the electro-retinogram (ERG) is usually markedly abnormal
   E topical antiviral medication is effective in treatment of rubella keratitis

41 With retinoblastoma,

   A the child often has a history of low birth weight
   B calcification is most suggestive of toxocariasis
   C the eye is often microphthalmic
   D most cases of hereditary retinoblastoma have a family history
   E the daughter of a mother who has had bilateral retinoblastomas has a 45% chance of having a retinoblastoma

42 In a patient with anterior ischaemic optic neuropathy (AION),

   A a normal erythrocyte sedimentation rate (ESR) excludes giant cell arteritis
   B hemianopic visual field loss is typical
   C patients with non-arteritic AION should have carotid Doppler studies performed
   D crowding of the optic disc may be a factor in the pathogenesis of non-arteritic AION
   E glaucoma is not associated with non-arteritic AION

43 In patients with benign intracranial hypertension,

   A there may be a VI nerve palsy
   B the CSF may contain increased protein
   C the visual field may show an enlarged blind spot
   D steroids can be a cause
   E transient 'blackouts' of vision may occur

44 Carotid artery disease is a cause of

   A iris neovascularization
   B a cholesterol embolus (Hollenhorst plaque)

C photopsia
D choroidal detachments
E Horner's syndrome

45 Regarding cranial nerve palsies,

A a painful III nerve palsy could be associated with diabetes
B an acoustic neuroma can cause loss of corneal sensation
C lid elevation on downgaze can occur after a III nerve palsy
D an acquired IV nerve palsy occurs most commonly as a result of a posterior fossa tumour
E giant cell arteritis can cause a VI nerve palsy

46 In a patient with optic neuritis,

A colour vision is often retained despite poor visual acuity
B a shortened P100 on visual evoked potential is consistent with the diagnosis
C a retinal vasculitis may suggest a diagnosis of multiple sclerosis
D four or more paraventricular lesions in the brain on MRI are suggestive of a diagnosis of multiple sclerosis
E oral steroid therapy may help prevent the onset of multiple sclerosis

47 Features of pseudopapilloedema, as a result of a buried optic nerve drusen, that are not found in true papilloedema are:

A absent central cup but retained spontaneous venous pulsation
B peripapillary retinal folds
C abnormal branching of vessels on the optic disc
D irregular disc margin with abnormality of peripapillary retinal pigment epithelium (RPE)
E marked fluorescein leakage from disc vessels

48 Features associated with neurofibromatosis type 1 include:

A Lisch nodules
B acoustic neuroma
C optic nerve glioma
D posterior subcapsular cataract
E sphenoid bone dysplasia

49 Regarding anisocoria,

   A when it becomes more pronounced in bright lighting conditions an abnormality of the smaller pupil is implied
   B when associated with vermiform movements of the sphincter it is likely to be due to Horner's syndrome
   C a miosed pupil is found in longstanding Holmes–Adie syndrome
   D the degree of physiological anisocoria may be more pronounced in low illumination
   E it can be caused by botulinum toxin

50 Causes of a pale optic disc include:

   A meningioma
   B Tay–Sachs disease
   C glaucoma
   D pan-retinal photocoagulation
   E retinitis pigmentosa

51 The following statements about AIDS-related illnesses are true:

   A optic neuritis may be caused by cytomegalovirus
   B HIV alone may cause meningitis
   C ocular toxoplasmosis is common in AIDS
   D herpes simplex typically results in posterior pole retinitis
   E progressive multifocal leucoencephalopathy is viral in origin

52 Features of myotonic dystrophy include:

   A pigmentary retinopathy
   B cardiomyopathy
   C insulin-resistant diabetes
   D ptosis
   E a tendency for venous thrombosis

53 Typical features of dorsal midbrain syndrome include:

   A impaired accommodation
   B convergence–retraction nystagmus

C impaired upgaze
D ptosis
E pupil constriction to light but not to near

54 Contrasting computerized tomography scanning (CT scan) and magnetic resonance imaging (MRI),

A with non-contrast MRI bright signal within vessels indicates blood flow
B MRI may display images in any anatomical plane
C CT has a faster image acquisition time
D CT provides better soft tissue definition
E MRI is contraindicated in those with amalgam fillings

55 Regarding the argon laser,

A it causes photodisruption
B it has peak wavelengths of 488 and 514 nm
C it may be used for peripheral iridotomy
D argon 'green' should be avoided near the macula
E it is used in cycloablation

56 Regarding drug toxicity and the eye,

A tamoxifen causes peripheral pigmentation
B thioridazine may cause an exudative maculopathy
C desferrioxamine may cause an optic neuropathy
D digoxin can affect colour vision
E canthaxanthine can cause a maculopathy

57 Regarding albinism,

A a subgroup may bleed excessively on teeth extraction
B oculocutaneous albinism is autosomal recessive
C 10% of fibres decussate at the chiasm
D myopic astigmatism is more common
E carriers of ocular albinism may have iris transillumination

58 The following are thought to be caused by herpes viruses:

   A acute retinal necrosis
   B progressive outer retinal necrosis
   C punctate inner choroidopathy
   D serpiginous choroiditis
   E multiple evanescent white dot syndrome

59 Regarding giant cells,

   A Touton giant cells occur in chalazia
   B foreign body giant cells may have randomly arranged nuclei
   C giant cells occur in leprosy
   D giant cells occur with caseating granulomata in sarcoidosis
   E Langerhans giant cells are seen with xanthogranulomas

60 Tumours originating in the ciliary body include:

   A medulloepithelioma
   B adenoma
   C adenocarcinoma
   D retinoblastoma
   E squamous cell carcinoma

PAPER 2

Questions

61 The following features of ptosis are correctly associated:

   A a congenital ptosis with a raised skin crease
   B an aponeurotic defect and good levator function
   C an overshoot of the lid when returning gaze from down to straight ahead in myasthenia gravis
   D 4 mm of ptosis and Horner's syndrome
   E lid elevation on moving the jaw and aberrant regeneration of the III nerve

62 Regarding nasolacrimal conditions,

   A an inflamed lacrimal sac mucocele should be drained through the skin if possible
   B a mid-common canalicular block may be due to herpetic disease
   C an infant with a watering eye should by syringed and probed at 6 months
   D a blockage of the nasolacrimal duct can be treated with a dacryocystorhinostomy
   E proximal common canalicular block may require a Lester Jones tube

63 In dysthyroid eye disease,

   A 50% of patients require surgery
   B reduced colour vision implies exposure keratopathy
   C the inferior rectus is the most commonly involved muscle
   D visual field constriction may occur
   E squint surgery should be carried out before correction of lid retraction

64 Periorbital capillary haemangiomas

   A are commonest in the superonasal quadrant of the orbit and upper lid
   B usually regress within the first year of life
   C when large may be associated with thrombocytopenia
   D are not associated with glaucoma
   E if complicated by amblyopia usually require surgery

65 In the management of an enlarged lacrimal gland,

   A a test for anti-neutrophil cytoplasmic antibodies (ANCAs) may be helpful
   B if a malignant tumour is suspected it should not be biopsied
   C a diagnosis of sarcoidosis should be considered
   D a malignant tumour has a good prognosis
   E a diagnosis of Behçet's disease should be considered

66 Causes of conjunctival cicatrization include:

   A linear IgA disease
   B graft versus host disease
   C Stevens–Johnson syndrome
   D thyroid eye disease
   E paraneoplastic syndrome

67 In patients with atopic eye disease,

   A Tranta's dots suggest giant papillary conjunctivitis
   B seasonal variation is a characteristic of adult atopic keratoconjunctivitis
   C keratoconus may be found
   D vernal keratoconjunctivitis generally has a good visual prognosis
   E serum IgE levels are elevated in vernal keratoconjunctivitis

68 Regarding corneal grafting,

   A small grafts are liable to more problems with astigmatism
   B large grafts are more likely to reject
   C using a donor button slightly larger than the host button increases astigmatism
   D HLA matching is routinely performed
   E it is less successful with vascularized host cornea

69 In chemical injuries,

   A detailed assessment of the extent of the injury must be carried out before beginning any treatment
   B topical steroids are contraindicated at all stages as they increase the risk of corneal perforation
   C topical ascorbic acid may assist in collagen repair

D   ammonia rapidly penetrates the cornea
E   acids typically result in more severe limbal ischaemia

70 In the differential diagnosis of peripheral corneal ulceration,

   A   a dellen is usually associated with reduced corneal sensation
   B   Terrien's degeneration is usually bilateral
   C   in staphylococcal hypersensitivity a clear zone usually separates the infiltrate from the limbus
   D   reduced corneal sensation may indicate herpetic disease
   E   Mooren's ulcer is usually associated with seropositive rheumatoid arthritis

71 In the diagnosis and management of corneal ulceration,

   A   chocolate agar is used to culture *Haemophilus*
   B   Rose-Bengal stains the base of a dendritic ulcer
   C   *Corynebacterium diphtheriae* can cause a corneal ulcer in the presence of a previously intact epithelium
   D   *Neisseria gonorrhoeae* is Gram positive
   E   *Pseudomonas* is usually sensitive to gentamicin

72 Keratoconus is associated with

   A   contact lens wear
   B   diabetes
   C   Crouzon's disease
   D   vernal catarrh
   E   a family history

73 When performing laser-assisted interstitial keratomileusis (LASIK),

   A   the intra-ocular pressure is raised to 65 mmHg
   B   the flap is hinged nasally
   C   the posterior surface of the cut flap is lasered
   D   the flap is closed with four cardinal sutures
   E   flap adhesion is confirmed by pressing on the corneal periphery

74 The following may be associated with cataract formation:

   A Wilson's disease
   B myasthenia gravis
   C retinitis pigmentosa
   D amyloidosis
   E hypocalcaemia

75 With regard to cataracts in children,

   A anterior polar cataracts usually cause marked visual impairment
   B posterior polar cataracts may be associated with capsular fragility
   C lamellar (zonular) cataracts are the most commonly found
   D congenital rubella results in posterior subcapsular cataracts
   E sutural cataracts rarely impair vision severely

76 Glaucoma secondary to trauma

   A occurs in 50% of patients with angle recession
   B is usually found in patients with high pressure immediately after trauma, which does not settle
   C may be due to ghost cells
   D can develop as a result of a lead intra-ocular foreign body
   E may be due to a cyclodialysis

77 On gonioscopy,

   A the Zeiss gonioscope is useful in diagnosing peripheral anterior synechiae
   B if the scleral spur can be seen 360° the angle is incapable of closure
   C inferior trabecular pigmentation is nearly always pathological
   D increased trabecular pigmentation is associated with the pseudoexfoliation syndrome
   E abnormal vessels can be seen in the angle with Fuch's heterochromic cyclitis

78 Regarding congenital glaucoma syndromes,

   A posterior embryotoxon is a feature of Axenfeld's syndrome
   B Rieger's syndrome is autosomal dominant

C   neurofibromatosis type II is associated with glaucoma, especially if there is a neurofibroma of the upper lid
D   primary congenital glaucoma is mainly X-linked
E   Haab's striae are classically circumlinear horizontal lines in Descemet's membrane

79 Regarding glaucoma surgery,

   A   acetazolamide can be helpful in treating a leaking bleb post-operatively
   B   Vicryl sutures should be used to enable post-operative argon suture lysis
   C   trabecular tissue must be removed for a trabeculectomy to work
   D   chronic hypotony is a risk factor for suprachoroidal haemorrhage
   E   hypotony can cause choroidal folds

80 Regarding ocular melanomas,

   A   epithelioid cell type has the best prognosis
   B   the nuclei of spindle B cells are more ovoid than spindle A
   C   a collar stud profile may develop when a melanoma breaks through Bruch's membrane
   D   they are the most common malignancy affecting the eye
   E   most iris melanomas have a spindle cell type

81 The following may be associated with iris heterochromia:

   A   siderosis
   B   multiple sclerosis
   C   Waardenberg's syndrome
   D   juvenile xanthogranuloma
   E   congenital Horner's syndrome

82 The following clinical findings are compatible with the diagnosis given:

   A   raised intra-ocular pressure (IOP) and a herpes-associated iritis
   B   a fibrinous uveitis and diabetes
   C   cystoid macular oedema and HLA B27-positive uveitis
   D   'mutton fat' keratic precipitates (KPs) in punctate inner choroidopathy (PIC)
   E   anterior uveitis and toxoplasmosis

83 The following systemic associations with conditions that can cause uveitis are correct:

   A oral and genital ulceration and sarcoidosis
   B deafness and Vogt–Koyanagi–Harada syndrome (VKH)
   C erythema nodosum and sarcoidosis
   D a swollen ankle and Reiter's syndrome
   E erythema nodosum and acute posterior multifocal placoid pigment epitheliopathy (APMPPE)

84 Angioid streaks

   A usually radiate from the macula
   B are generally hypofluorescent in the early stages of fluorescein angiography
   C predispose to choroidal rupture in blunt trauma
   D may be associated with sickle cell anaemia
   E predispose to choroidal neovascularization

85 Features found in central serous chorioretinopathy include:

   A a visible choroidal neovascular membrane
   B the symptom of micropsia
   C mottled appearance of the retinal pigment epithelium
   D intense early leakage on fluorescein angiography
   E prodromal viral illness in 50%

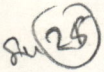

86 Regarding argon laser treatment of diabetic retinopathy,

   A treatment should be given for exudate without oedema near the fovea
   B a circinate should be treated two disc diameters from the fovea
   C patients with new vessels at the disc covering more than one-third of the disc area have a 10% chance of going blind in 2 years
   D 500 burns are usually adequate for pan-retinal photocoagulation
   E pan-retinal photocoagulation may make macular oedema worse

87 Regarding diabetic retinopathy,

   A venous beading is a preproliferative change
   B the presence of cotton wool spots can suggest additional hypertension or renal disease

C retinopathy usually improves in pregnancy
D with the introduction of good diabetic control retinopathy may initially get worse
E intraretinal microvascular abnormalities (IRMAs) are found with background retinopathy

88 The following are true about sickle cell retinopathy:

A angioid streaks can occur
B patches of iris atrophy are a recognized feature
C salmon patches are indicative of choroidal neovascularization
D black sunbursts are peripheral chorioretinal scars
E pan-retinal photocoagulation may be required

89 The following may cause progressive night blindness:

A fundus albipunctatus
B choroideraemia
C vitamin A deficiency
D Oguchi disease
E Goldman–Favre syndrome

90 With chloroquine (CQ) and hydroxychloroquine (HCQ) therapy,

A irreversible corneal crystalline deposits may occur
B a bull's-eye maculopathy may occur
C early retinopathy is characterized by absence of the foveal reflex and granular pigmentary changes at the macula
D corneal changes are not associated with an increased risk of maculopathy
E retinopathy detected by Amsler grid testing may be reversible

91 In Stargardt's disease the following are true:

A a dark choroid may be found on fluorescein angiography
B the retinal blood vessels become narrow early in the disease process
C if retinal flecks are present they leak fluorescein
D the peripheral fields are full
E onset usually occurs before 20 years of age

92 Retinal arterial occlusions are associated with

   A atrial myxoma
   B homocystinuria
   C acute retinal necrosis
   D giant cell arteritis
   E Wilson's disease

93 The following diets may be helpful:

   A a phytanic acid-free diet in Refsum's disease
   B vitamin E supplements in abetalipoproteinaemia
   C a low protein diet in choroideraemia
   D vitamin B6 supplements in gyrate atrophy
   E vitamin A in Stickler's syndrome

94 Regarding toxicity of intra-ocular foreign bodies,

   A zinc causes chronic chalcosis
   B pure iron is inert
   C aluminium leads to a severe inflammatory reaction
   D sunflower cataract is a feature of chronic chalcosis
   E in siderosis, ERG b-wave amplitude is characteristically reduced

95 Indications for vitrectomy in rhegmatogenous retinal detachment include:

   A giant retinal tears
   B fibrovascular proliferation
   C traumatic dialysis
   D macular breaks
   E posterior vitreous detachment

96 In the differential diagnosis of rhegmatogenous retinal detachment the following statements are true:

   A exudative detachments are limited by the vortex vein exit sites
   B retinoschisis is usually bilateral and superotemporal
   C 'tobacco dust' in the vitreous suggests a retinal break
   D choroidal detachment may co-exist with retinal detachment
   E traction retinal detachment usually requires urgent surgical repair

97 Regarding vertical squints,

   A a positive Bielschowsky head-tilt test, in a patient with a superior oblique palsy, involves the paretic eye elevating on head tilt away from the side of the lesion
   B surgery to decrease a hyperdeviation after a IV nerve palsy may involve inferior oblique recession on the same side
   C an upshoot of the eye may occur on adduction in Brown's syndrome
   D superior oblique over action commonly occurs with an esotropia
   E a base-down prism bar can be used to measure a hypertropia

98 Associations of Duane's syndrome include:

   A Goldenhar's syndrome
   B Klippel–Feil syndrome
   C heterochromia iridis
   D deafness
   E colobomata

99 Regarding abnormal head postures,

   A a face turn to the right suggests a left VI nerve palsy
   B a chin-down head tilt to the right and face turn to the right suggest a right IV nerve palsy
   C an abnormal head posture is not uncommon in nystagmus
   D unilateral deafness can cause an abnormal head posture
   E patients with thyroid eye disease not uncommonly develop a chin-up posture

100 Features found in congenital esotropia include:

   A onset at 4 months of age
   B asymmetrical optokinetic nystagmus
   C dissociated vertical deviation (DVD)
   D skew deviation
   E latent nystagmus

101 Regarding aniridia,

   A glaucoma is typically present from birth
   B zonular support is often abnormal
   C cycloplegia is not required for refraction in young children
   D peripheral anterior synechiae and corneal endothelial ingrowth into the drainage angle may be progressive
   E inherited cases are frequently associated with bilateral Wilms' tumour

102 The following statements about ophthalmia neonatorum are true:

   A routine prophylaxis with silver nitrate 1% is used in the UK
   B chlamydial conjunctivitis usually begins within 2 days of birth
   C gonococcal conjunctivitis may lead to a perforating keratitis
   D topical acyclovir is used as monotherapy in herpes simplex ophthalmia
   E a Gram-negative cocco-bacillus on Gram stain usually indicates *Haemophilus* infection

103 In a child with cloudy cornea at birth the following features are found:

   A a central opacity in corneal dermoid
   B a corneal diameter of 9 mm in congenital glaucoma
   C bilateral involvement in congenital hereditary endothelial dystrophy (CHED)
   D raised intra-ocular pressure in Hurler's syndrome
   E corneal diameter is normal in CHED

104 The following tests may be abnormal/positive in giant cell arteritis:

   A serum von Willebrand factor levels
   B C-reactive protein (CRP) levels
   C temporal artery biopsy after 48 hours of systemic steroids
   D full blood count
   E protein electrophoresis

105 In Horner's syndrome,

   A the pupil does not react to light
   B long-standing cases are associated with heterochromia
   C decreased facial sweating suggests that the causative lesion is distal to the superior cervical ganglion

D adrenaline 1:1000 will not dilate a preganglionic Horner's
E the pupil demonstrates tonic vermiform movements

106 The following eponymous clinical phenomena are correctly associated:

A L'Hermitte's sign is an 'electric shock' sensation down the back on neck flexion in a patient with multiple sclerosis
B Uhthoff's phenomenon is the sensation of seeing a pendulum swing in a three-dimensional way, i.e. in a circle, when it is only swinging in one plane
C Pulfrich's phenomenon is the worsening of symptoms of multiple sclerosis on getting into a hot bath
D Cogan's lid twitch and myasthenia gravis
E Anton's syndrome is the denial of visual loss

107 In fourth nerve palsy,

A a vertical fusion range less than 3 dioptres suggests a congenital palsy
B the hyperdeviation increases on contralateral gaze
C men are more frequently affected
D bilateral palsies should always be suspected in traumatic cases
E microvascular occlusion is the most common cause

108 About the swollen optic disc,

A in optic neuritis visual acuity usually improves by 6 weeks
B optic neuritis in children is more commonly bilateral than in adults
C visual acuity is usually reduced with papilloedema
D an altitudinal field defect is typical for an anterior ischaemic optic neuropathy
E eye movement is often painful with an arteritic anterior ischaemic optic neuropathy

109 The following visual field defects are correctly associated:

A anterior ischaemic optic neuropathy characteristically causes a central scotoma
B papilloedema can mimic bitemporal hemianopia
C a bilateral centrocaecal scotoma can occur with a basilar artery embolus
D a superior bitemporal quadrantinopia occurs with craniopharyngiomas
E an occipital lobe tumour is more likely to produce a congruous homonomous hemianopia than an anterior parietal lobe lesion

110 Features of neurofibromatosis include:

   A subungual fibromas
   B brushfield spots
   C 50% of the siblings of a patient may have signs
   D optic nerve glioma developing in childhood
   E retinal astrocytic hamartomas

111 In ocular myasthenia gravis,

   A early surgical correction of ptosis is indicated
   B vertically acting extra-ocular muscles are most commonly affected
   C anti-acetylcholine receptor antibodies are found in about 50%
   D anisocoria is a common feature
   E electrophysiology is characteristic

112 Optic neuropathy may be caused by

   A vitamin D deficiency
   B rifampicin
   C methanol
   D lead toxicity
   E ethambutol

113 The following conditions may be worsened during pregnancy:

   A pituitary adenoma
   B keratoconus
   C meningioma
   D uveal melanoma
   E diabetic retinopathy

114 Features of mitochondrial myopathies include:

   A ptosis as the first feature
   B diplopia commonly
   C exposure keratopathy
   D the risk of heart block in some patients
   E 'ragged-red' fibres on electron microscopy studies of muscle biopsy

Paper 2 *Questions* 27

115 The following statements about disordered visual perception are true:

   A Charles Bonnet syndrome may occur after optic tract infarction
   B isolated alexia may be caused by a large left occipital lesion
   C alexia with agraphia occurs with left parietal lesions
   D visual neglect often occurs with right parietal lesions
   E visual agnosia may be caused by bilateral inferior occipital lesions

116 Possible adverse effects of pan-retinal photocoagulation include:

   A alteration of colour vision in the therapist
   B central scotoma
   C impaired night vision
   D constriction of peripheral visual fields below the driving standard
   E rhegmatogenous retinal detachment

117 Iris neovascularization

   A can be treated by pan-retinal photocoagulation
   B may be secondary to carotid artery stenosis
   C can occur in Coat's disease
   D usually starts in the angle
   E invariably causes glaucoma

118 Regarding electrodiagnostics,

   A the electro-oculogram (EOG) originates in the retinal pigment epithelium
   B the 'a'-wave of the electro-retinogram (ERG) originates in Muller cells
   C the pattern ERG is a measure of macular function
   D a delayed visual evoked potential (VEP) p-wave may be found with optic neuritis
   E 110% is an abnormal EOG Arden index

119 In eyelid pathology,

   A cellular atypia in solar keratosis is usually found in the dermis
   B basal cell carcinoma may contain keratotic whorls
   C basal cell carcinoma originates in the basal cells of the epidermis
   D a chalazion may contain giant cells
   E a chalazion may contain fat vacuoles

120 In the pathology of macular degeneration,

    A Bruch's membrane is thinner than normal
    B drusen are deposits of PAS-positive material beneath the retinal pigment epithelium
    C subretinal neovascularization starts from the choroid
    D Bruch's membrane may have breaks in it
    E vitreous haemorrhage can occur

Paper 3

Questions

121 Comparing the features of acquired aponeurotic with congenital dystrophic ptosis,

    A in aponeurotic ptosis the skin crease is elevated
    B Fasanella Servat operation (tarso-conjunctival excision) may be suitable for mild congenital ptosis
    C levator function is reduced in aponeurotic ptosis
    D lid lag occurs in dystrophic ptosis
    E the skin crease may be absent in dystrophic ptosis

122 When investigating the lacrimal outflow system,

    A a positive Jones primary test implies physiological functioning of the system
    B absence of fluorescein in the nose but patency to saline in the Jones secondary test implies a canalicular or punctal stenosis
    C scintillography is useful in those found to be blocked on syringing
    D a 'soft stop' is characteristic of a mucocele
    E a dacryocystogram demonstrates the anatomy proximal to an obstruction

123 In an adult with proptosis

    A a mucocele causes axial proptosis
    B dysthyroid eye disease is the commonest cause
    C lymphoid tumours commonly show bony erosion on CT scan
    D an optic nerve sheath meningioma is most frequently found in middle aged women
    E cavernous haemangiomata are commonest in young adults

124 Signs strongly suggestive of an orbital blow-out fracture include:

    A periorbital oedema
    B a fluid level in the ipsilateral maxillary sinus on plain X-ray

C infra-orbital hypoaesthesia
D limitation of vertical eye movements
E surgical emphysema of the eyelids

125 Orbital cellulitis

A most commonly occurs as a result of sphenoidal sinusitis
B is most commonly due to *Haemophilus influenzae* in a child
C should have CT scanning of the orbit and sinuses performed in most cases
D can cause a central retinal artery occlusion
E can cause a cavernous sinus thrombosis

126 Scleritis

A in the form of scleromalacia perforans is painful
B is associated with Wegener's granulomatosis
C can cause choroidal folds
D can occur in association with herpes zoster ophthalmicus
E can cause uveitis

127 The following are features of vernal keratoconjunctivitis:

A itching
B Tranta's dots
C giant papillae (cobblestone)
D pseudogerontoxon
E symblepharon

128 With regard to corneal dystrophies,

A Reis–Buckler's dystrophy presents with blurred vision in middle age
B macular dystrophy has an autosomal recessive inheritance pattern
C lattice dystrophy frequently causes recurrent erosions
D granular dystrophy causes progressive corneal oedema
E Meesman's dystrophy affects the endothelium

129 In the investigation of dry eye,

A a positive anti Ro/ss-A antibody is consistent with primary Sjögren's syndrome

B the normal tear film break-up time is less than 10 s
C basal and reflex tear secretion is measured by the Schirmer test after administration of topical benoxinate
D punctal epithelial erosions are commonest in the interpalpebral conjunctiva
E staining with Rose-Bengal causes discomfort

130 Peripheral corneal ulceration

A in marginal keratitis starts as a subepithelial infiltrate
B in acne rosacea is associated with peripheral vascularization
C as a result of a Mooren's ulcer classically has an undermined edge at the periphery
D may be associated with scleritis
E is a feature of hypersensitivity to eyelid flora

131 The following corneal pigment depositions are correctly associated:

A Stocker's line with pterygium
B Ferry's line with a trabeculectomy
C Hudson–Stahli line with amiodarone
D Kayser–Fleischer ring in keratoconus
E chrysiasis caused by gold therapy

132 With keratoconus,

A Fleischer's ring is a feature
B corneal nerves are often prominent
C acute hydrops is more common in Down's syndrome patients
D inferior steepening is seen on corneal topography
E hypermetropia is common

133 The following types of cataracts and their associations are correctly linked:

A myotonic dystrophy and 'oil-droplet' cataracts
B posterior subcapsular cataracts and uveitis
C nuclear cataract and systemic corticosteroid treatment
D severe alkali injury and cortical cataract
E anterior subcapsular cataracts and atopic dermatitis

134 The following are recognized to be associated with increased risk of failure of trabeculectomy:

    A previous uncomplicated cataract surgery
    B diabetes
    C prolonged topical glaucoma medication
    D neovascular glaucoma
    E patient age over 70

135 Regarding aqueous dynamics,

    A intra-ocular pressure (IOP) is highest in the morning
    B 80% of aqueous is produced by active secretion
    C a retinal detachment can cause ciliary body shutdown and so a decrease in aqueous production
    D the uveoscleral route accounts for 40% of outflow
    E pilocarpine increases uveoscleral outflow

136 With the pigment dispersion syndrome,

    A the anterior chamber tends to be shallow
    B pigment granules are found on the surface of the iris
    C pilocarpine is potentially a good first line of treatment if glaucoma develops
    D young black males are the most commonly affected
    E corneal oedema and haloes can occur

137 Regarding secondary glaucomas,

    A ghost cell glaucoma occurs in phakic eyes
    B irido-corneal endothelial syndromes are usually bilateral
    C raised pressure following pan-retinal photocoagulation can develop as a result of increased episcleral pressure
    D Sturge–Weber syndrome is associated with angle-closure glaucoma
    E melanocytic glaucoma is due to tumour cells invading the trabecular meshwork

138 In the drug treatment of open-angle glaucoma,

    A betaxolol is a safe first line of treatment in asthmatics
    B latanoprost increases uveoscleral outflow

C   acetazolamide can prolong the action of warfarin
D   pilocarpine should be used cautiously in aphakic glaucoma
E   apraclonidine is a prostaglandin inhibitor

139 Ultrasound findings consistent with uveal melanoma include:

   A   high internal reflectivity
   B   choroidal excavation
   C   evidence of internal vascularity
   D   typically a lobular surface to the lesion
   E   extra-scleral extension

140 Regarding endophthalmitis,

   A   it most commonly presents in the first 24 hours after cataract surgery
   B   if it occurs a few months after cataract surgery, it is usually due to *Staphylococcus aureus*
   C   treatment should include intravitreal gentamicin
   D   following a trabeculectomy it is more common if mitomycin is used
   E   it has a poor prognosis if due to *Streptococcus*

141 In Fuch's heterochromic cyclitis,

   A   Koeppe nodules may be seen
   B   a hyphaema may develop during cataract surgery
   C   vitreous cells occur
   D   iris transillumination is a feature
   E   posterior synechiae occur

142 Retinal haemorrhages

   A   in non-accidental injury may be associated with a subdural haematoma
   B   can occur in asphyxia
   C   can be associated with vitamin K deficiency
   D   may be induced by high altitude
   E   occur in choroideraemia

143 Possible causes of choroidal neovascularization include:

 A optic disc drusen
 B argon retinal photocoagulation
 C toxoplasmosis
 D posterior vitreous detachment
 E choroidal naevus

144 Regarding central serous chorioretinopathy,

 A it is more common in men
 B there may be widespread leaking points on indocyanine green
 C visual acuity can often be improved with a +1-dioptre lens
 D focal argon laser treatment is sometimes used
 E it can be found in association with an optic disc pit

145 With regard to diabetic retinopathy,

 A 50% of diabetic patients have retinopathy after 7–10 years
 B 25% of the diabetic population have some form of retinopathy
 C the probability of progression from preproliferative to proliferative retinopathy is 50% over 2 years
 D 5% of the diabetic population have proliferative retinopathy
 E the incidence of proliferative diabetic retinopathy after 25 years is 25%

146 The following are true of sickle cell (SC) retinopathy:

 A SC trait is found in about 8% of the black population
 B SS (homozygous) disease is found in less than 1% of the black population
 C retinopathy is most severe in SS disease
 D SC disease is found in less than 0.5% of the black population
 E retinopathy is found in SC trait

147 The following causes of retinitis pigmentosa may also cause deafness:

 A Refsum's syndrome
 B Usher's syndrome
 C Kearn–Sayre syndrome
 D Alstrom's syndrome
 E Bardet–Biedl syndrome

148 Causes of macular exudate include:

A radiation retinopathy
B von Hippel–Lindau disease
C Coat's disease
D Stargardt's macular dystrophy
E branch retinal vein occlusion

149 Regarding central retinal vein occlusions (CRVOs),

A a relative afferent pupil defect is expected if it is ischaemic
B a young patient has a better prognosis
C aspirin should be avoided with an acute CRVO
D fundus fluorescein angiography is necessary for diagnosis if they are ischaemic
E they are more common in men

150 Regarding fluorescein angiography,

A fluorescein can cause a false-positive urine glucose test
B the first phase of the angiogram is the arterial phase
C it takes 15 s for the dye to reach the retinal circulation
D late staining of the disc is pathological
E anaphylactic shock should be treated with 1 mL of 1:10 000 adrenaline, intramuscularly

151 Retinal vasculitis

A may cause sheathing of retinal blood vessels
B can cause retinal neovascularization
C causes fluorescein to leak from retinal blood vessels
D occurs in multiple sclerosis
E in sarcoidosis mainly involves the arteries

152 The following abnormalities are expected in the carriers of these diseases:

A a subnormal EOG in Best's disease
B iris transillumination in X-linked ocular albinism
C peripheral retinal pigment epithelial atrophy in choroideraemia

D nystagmus in cone dystrophy
E maculopathy in Stargardt's disease

153 With respect to macular holes,

A retinal detachment rarely occurs
B involvement of the second eye is rare
C vitrectomy is indicated for stage 1 holes
D in stage 4 holes posterior vitreous detachment is always present
E an operculum may be seen

154 The following are associated with increased risk of retinal detachment:

A uncomplicated extracapsular cataract surgery
B traumatic hyphaema
C homocystinuria
D lattice degeneration
E AIDS

155 Retinoschisis

A is usually superonasal
B may have a pigmented demarcation line
C may have white dots on the inner limiting membrane
D may cause a visual field defect
E is more common in myopic patients

156 In the management of childhood strabismus,

A full hypermetropic correction should be given to a child with an exotropia
B a VI nerve palsy is part of the differential of an esotropia
C the squint should be corrected before amblyopia treatment
D congenital esotropias have a good prognosis for binocular single vision
E an esotropia for near could be associated with a high AC/A ratio

157 Regarding exotropias,

A any degree of myopia should be corrected
B amblyopia is a frequent association

C 'A' patterns are commonly associated with distance exotropia
D a consecutive exotropia can occur spontaneously
E the use of a +3-dioptre lens in conjunction with a cover test helps distinguish between a simulated and true divergence excess

158 The following are medical contraindications to corneal donation:

A recipients of pituitary hormone
B previous intra-ocular surgery
C congenital rubella
D optic nerve glioma
E Hodgkin's lymphoma

159 With regard to refraction in infants,

A the mean refractive error in the newborn is emmetropia
B hypermetropia may be overestimated on retinoscopy
C Leber's amaurosis is associated with myopia
D astigmatism is usually against-the-rule
E tropicamide 1% should be instilled 1 hour before refraction

160 In a child with retinitis pigmentosa (RP),

A severe visual loss suggests autosomal dominant inheritance
B EOG testing often shows pronounced abnormalities in infancy
C ERG typically shows a reduction in both rod and cone signals
D dietary manipulation is of benefit in some forms
E reduced visual acuity may result from cystoid macular oedema

161 With regard to retinopathy of prematurity (ROP),

A babies born under 31 weeks' gestational age should be screened
B threshold ROP is estimated to have a 50% risk of blindness
C 50% of babies < 1500 g develop stage 3 ROP
D the mean age for onset of threshold disease is 37 weeks post-menstrual age (PMA)
E stage 3 disease is an elevated line of retinal neovascularization

162 The following statements about proptosis in childhood are true:

A rapid onset suggests rhabdomyosarcoma
B orbital tumours are the most common cause of proptosis
C neuroblastoma deposits are commonly bilateral
D bony abnormalities are best seen on MRI
E *café-au-lait* spots suggest a diagnosis of a dermoid cyst

163 The following can be symptoms or signs of temporal arteritis:

A jaw claudication
B angina
C temporal scalp necrosis
D erythema nodosum
E nail-bed splinter haemorrhages

164 The uses of the optokinetic nystagmus (OKN) drum include:

A differentiating true blindness from hysterical blindness
B differentiating between a visual pathway lesion in the parietal or occipital lobes
C demonstrating convergence retraction nystagmus
D assessing whether an esotropia was congenital
E detecting a temporal lobe lesion

165 Regarding myasthenia gravis,

A it may present with ocular features only
B single-fibre electromyography (EMG) is an appropriate test
C a tensilon test may be negative
D the cerebrospinal fluid may be abnormal
E it can masquerade as an oculomotor palsy

166 Regarding carotico-cavernous fistulae,

A the most common cause of visual loss is open-angle glaucoma
B the shunt should always be closed
C they usually occur traumatically
D MRI may show enlarged extra-ocular muscles
E MRI may show a dilated superior ophthalmic vein

Paper 3 *Questions* 39

167 The following statements about optic disc drusen are true:

- **A** inheritance may be autosomal dominant
- **B** extensive visual field loss may be present
- **C** angioid streaks are associated
- **D** they are commonest in dark-skinned races
- **E** retinitis pigmentosa may be associated

168 Herpes zoster ophthalmicus can cause

- **A** optic neuritis
- **B** a stroke
- **C** a dendritic keratitis
- **D** chickenpox in a contact
- **E** ptosis

169 The following features are associated with type 2 neurofibromatosis:

- **A** presenile posterior subcapsular cataract
- **B** Lisch nodules
- **C** acoustic neuroma
- **D** optic nerve glioma
- **E** *café-au-lait* spots

170 In essential blepharospasm,

- **A** spasm does not occur during sleep
- **B** the pathogenesis involves chronic facial nerve root compression
- **C** men are more commonly affected
- **D** botulinum toxin injections are the treatment of choice
- **E** functional blindness may be caused

171 Possible causes of a relative afferent pupil defect (RAPD) include:

- **A** parietal lobe infarction
- **B** macular disciform scar
- **C** cataract
- **D** branch retinal artery occlusion
- **E** retrobulbar neuritis

172 The following ocular conditions are more common during pregnancy:

   A   scleritis
   B   retinal detachment
   C   optic neuritis
   D   central serous chorioretinopathy
   E   hypertensive retinopathy

173 Regarding nystagmus,

   A   congenital nystagmus secondary to visual loss clinically appears pendular
   B   in congenital nystagmus visual acuity may be better for near than for distance
   C   spasmus nutans has a poor prognosis
   D   opsoclonus can be a presenting sign of a neuroblastoma
   E   with cerebellar damage, nystagmus occurs towards the side of the lesion

174 When using a contact lens for retinal laser treatment,

   A   the Goldman standard three-mirror lens doubles the spot diameter on the retina
   B   a 500-µm burn is generally used in argon prophylactic pan-retinal photocoagulation (PRP)
   C   the Mainster Ultrafield lens reduces the spot size
   D   a 50-µm burn is generally used for focal macular treatment
   E   the Volk Quadraspheric lens almost doubles the spot size

175 The following are part of the visual standards for driving a car in the UK:

   A   being able to read a numberplate at 35 yards
   B   minimum horizontal visual field of 150°
   C   having normal colour vision
   D   monocular vision should be notified to the licensing centre
   E   an inferior homonymous quandrantanopia is not permitted

176 The following laser settings are appropriate:

   A   10 mJ energy for yttrium aluminium garnet (YAG) capsulotomy
   B   500 µm, 50 mW and 0.1 s for argon laser trabeculoplasty

C 500 μm, 200 mW and 0.2 s for argon PRP
D 3 mJ at three pulses per burst for YAG iridotomy
E 100 μm, 100 mW and 0.15 s for argon macular grid

177 Conditions associated with myopic refraction include:

A neonatal visual deprivation
B retinopathy of prematurity
C Stickler's syndrome
D gyrate atrophy
E albinism

178 The following are autosomal dominant:

A Best's disease
B Stargardt's
C Usher's syndrome
D juvenile retinoschisis
E Stickler's syndrome

179 The differential of a limbal tumour may include:

A a dermoid tumour
B squamous cell carcinoma
C basal cell carcinoma
D neurofibroma
E melanoma

180 Regarding pigmented lesions,

A pigmentation with a naevus of Ota may include a dark choroid
B primary acquired melanosis can be precancerous
C conjunctival naevi may have a junctional pattern
D conjunctival naevi occur most commonly at the limbus
E episcleral melanosis is precancerous

Paper 1

Answers

1   **A** = False   **B** = False   **C** = True   **D** = True   **E** = True

Keratoacanthoma is a rapidly growing benign ulcerating keratotic lesion that closely resembles squamous cell carcinoma. Resolution frequently occurs within 4–6 months. However, if there is any doubt about the diagnosis an excisional biopsy should be performed.

Basal cell carcinomas are the most common form of eyelid tumour. Those located in the medial canthal area or vertical midline of the face are much more likely to be deeply infiltrating and should be excised rather than treated by other means. Recurrent or atypical chalazia should be biopsied to exclude sebaceous cell carcinoma.

2   **A** = False   **B** = True   **C** = False   **D** = True   **E** = False

Basal cell carcinoma (BCC) is the commonest malignant tumour of the eyelids and is found in decreasing order of frequency on the lower lid, medial canthus, upper lid and lateral canthus. In xeroderma pigmentosum there is a defect of repair of damaged DNA. Areas exposed to ultraviolet radiation have an increased frequency of actinic related tumours.

The nodular type of BCC shows peripheral pallisading of the basal cells, whereas the morpheiform type shows radiating cords of basal cells with fibrotic changes of the surrounding stroma.

BCCs treated by radiotherapy and cryotherapy have higher recurrence rates and these treatment modalities should be avoided in the canthal areas where deep invasion is a risk.

Mohs' micrographic surgery is designed to preserve as much tissue as possible since sequential excision is guided by the presence of residual tumour on frozen section histology.

3   **A** = True   **B** = False   **C** = True   **D** = False   **E** = True

Causes of **acquired canalicular obstruction** include:

- **trauma**
- **viral infections**, herpes simplex and zoster

- **toxic medication** – **systemic** – idoxuridine
  5-fluorouracil
  – **topical** – phospholine iodide
- **autoimmune disorders,** pemphigoid
- **Stevens–Johnson syndrome**
- **iatrogenic,** traumatic lacrimal probing.

4 **A** = True **B** = False **C** = True **D** = True **E** = True

In assessing proptosis the following features are helpful: unilateral or bilateral, axial or non-axial, a palpable lesion, associated ocular features, restriction of eye movements, a bruit and signs of systemic disease. Thyroid disease is the commonest cause of proptosis whether unilateral or bilateral.

5 **A** = True **B** = True **C** = False **D** = True **E** = True

Enucleation should be performed rather than **evisceration** in eyes with known or suspected intra-ocular malignancy and severely traumatized eyes where complete removal of uveal tissue is desirable. Evisceration is preferable in endophthalmitis to avoid spread of infection to the orbit.

Removal of an eye in childhood results in reduced growth of the orbit unless the orbital volume is maintained by an adequate implant. A 20- to 22-mm adult-sized sphere implant should be used if possible.

Implant materials may be classified as

- **inert,** e.g. methyl methacrylate, silicone, acrylic
- **bioreactive,** e.g. hydroxyapatite, porous polyethylene.

Hydroxyapatite may be drilled 6–9 months post-operatively to allow placement of a prosthesis peg. Early exposure may be increased with this material, however. Inert spherical implants have low extrusion rates and are comfortable, but give poorer prosthesis motility.

Prostheses may be fitted within 4–8 weeks of eye removal.

6 **A** = False **B** = True **C** = False **D** = True **E** = False

Haemophilus influenzae is commonly responsible for **orbital and preseptal cellulitis** in children under the age of 5. The cellulitis usually originates from another infective source (e.g. otitis media) via haematogenous spread. Young children with orbital cellulitis should be hospitalized, with blood cultures taken to guide antibiotic therapy.

		Preseptal	Orbital
Route of infection		Inoculation through skin (+ haematogenous)	Spread from sinuses (+ haematogenous)
Lid involvement		Severe	Moderate/severe
Globe involvement		Absent	Involved
Vision		Normal	May be reduced (danger sign)
Ocular movements		Normal	May be reduced, painful

7   **A** = False   **B** = True   **C** = False   **D** = False   **E** = True

Factors affecting the outcome of **astigmatic keratotomy** include:

- **patient age,** wound healing is less good in older patients so overcorrection is more likely;
- **optical zone size,** incisions closer to the centre of the cornea result in far greater effect;
- **number of incisions**, single pairs of incisions result in 1:1 coupling (for each dioptre of flattening created in one meridian there is a corresponding dioptre of steepening at 90°). Spherical equivalence is not affected. Multiple incisions result in greater corneal instability and are more likely to induce irregular astigmatism;
- **incision length,** in general incisions should extend for no more than 90° (incisions are curved and parallel to the limbus);
- **incision depth,** incisions should be the maximum possible depth without causing perforation. Ideally a pachymeter should be used to measure corneal thickness preoperatively.

Contraindications (absolute and relative) include:
- keratoconus or other corneal ectasias
- corneal thinning due to other causes
- severe ocular surface disease
- unrealistic patient expectation
- high risk of blunt trauma (e.g. occupational risk).

8   **A** = True   **B** = False   **C** = False   **D** = False   **E** = True

Both class 1 and 2 MHC antigens are found in the cornea. **Allograft rejection** is mediated via T (CD4$^+$ and CD8$^+$) lymphocytes either via direct recognition of donor antigens or indirectly via antigen presentation. Rejection may occur at the epithelial, stromal or endothelial level. Tissue typing has not been definitively shown to improve graft survival rates in high-risk cases. Large grafts have increased risk of rejection. However, small grafts have increased problems because of astigmatism and may fail because of an inadequate number of endothelial cells transplanted.

Paper 1 Answers

Early graft failure (within 10 days) is caused by factors such as infection, uncontrolled uveitis, glaucoma, surgical trauma, primary endothelial failure and vitreous endothelial touch. Allograft rejection is a later phenomenon.

9   **A** = False   **B** = False   **C** = True   **D** = True   **E** = False

Macular dystrophy causes visual impairment early in life, lattice by about 30 years and granular may never cause severe impairment of vision. In some cases of Schnyder's corneal dystrophy a low-cholesterol diet may help.

10   **A** = True   **B** = True   **C** = True   **D** = True   **E** = False

Aetiology of **dry eye**

- **aqueous deficiency**
    idiopathic
    primary Sjögren's syndrome
    secondary Sjögren's syndrome (e.g. with rheumatoid arthritis, systemic lupus erythematosus, polyarteritis nodosa, Wegener's)
    Riley–Day syndrome (familial dysautonomia)
    neuroparalytic
    lacrimal gland infiltration (e.g. sarcoidosis, tumour)
    surgery in superotemporal fornix
    post-radiotherapy to lacrimal gland
- **drug-induced** (e.g. oral contraceptive pill, antihistamines, beta-blockers, phenothiazines, atropine)
- **mucin deficiency**
    conjunctival scarring (Stevens–Johnson syndrome, chemical burns, cicatricial pemphigoid)
    vitamin A deficiency
- **lipid deficiency**
    meibomian gland disease/blepharitis.

11   **A** = False   **B** = True   **C** = True   **D** = True   **E** = True

Salzman's nodular degeneration develops following chronic keratitis, trachoma or phlyctenulosis. Sodium versenate is a topical treatment for **band-shaped keratopathy**. It is applied to the corneal surface after epithelial debridement. Excimer laser has also been successfully used to remove band-shaped keratopathy.

Measures to prevent recurrence of **pterygium** include: conjunctival grafting, intra-operative application of mitomycin C or beta-irradiation, or post-operative mitomycin C drops.

Causes of a **filamentary keratitis** include: dry eye, neurotrophic keratopathy and superior limbic keratitis as well as prolonged patching.

12 **A** = False **B** = False **C** = True **D** = True **E** = True

***Acanthamoeba* keratitis** classically occurs in soft contact lens wearers, especially if tap water has come into contact with the lenses or case. Various species of *Acanthamoeba* are found in swimming pools, water supplies and soil. Keratitis may occur after superficial corneal trauma and concurrent exposure to an infective source. Initially, the diagnosis is often confused with herpetic keratitis as a pseudodendritic pattern of epithelial keratitis may be seen. This may also show a partial response to topical antivirals. Perineural infiltrates are very suggestive of the diagnosis. Pain is often disproportionately severe compared with the clinical findings. With severe *Acanthamoeba* keratitis a corneal ring infiltrate, hypopyon, glaucoma, hyphaema and cataract, as well as scleritis may be seen. *Acanthamoeba* can be cultured on a 'lawn' of *E. coli* or other coliforms spread on nutrient-free agar. Sometimes a corneal biopsy is required to make the diagnosis. The organisms may be identified by immunohistochemistry staining or stains such as calcofluor white.

13 **A** = False **B** = True **C** = False **D** = True **E** = True

Causes of **subluxated lenses** include:

- **inherited**
    Marfan's
    homocystinuria
    Weill–Marchesani syndrome
    sulphite oxidase deficiency
    Ehlers–Danlos syndrome
    familial ectopia lentis
    aniridia
    ectopia lentis et pupillae
- **acquired**
    trauma (probably the commonest cause in adults)
    buphthalmos
    pseudoexfoliation syndrome
    hypermature cataract
    high myopia
    syphilis (acquired).

Subluxation of the lens occurs in 60–80% of those with Marfan's and is usually superior. Accommodation is usually preserved as the zonules are elongated rather than broken. Only 7.5% progress to full dislocation. In homocystinuria the dislocation is usually inferior and the zonules break. Urinary sodium nitroprusside testing is usually positive, although urinary homocystine level testing is a more reliable diagnostic test. Patients have an increased risk of thromboembolic episodes. Forty to fifty per cent show some improvement on pyridoxine supplements.

14 **A** = True **B** = False **C** = False **D** = True **E** = False

Cystoid macular oedema reflects an increase in perifoveal capillary permeability, although the exact pathogenesis is unknown. The incidence is highest after intracapsular surgery and increases with perioperative complications. The peak incidence is 6–10 weeks post-operatively. Angiographic CMO is much more common than clinically evident CMO. Spontaneous resolution occurs in 95%. Lamellar holes may develop in severe cases.

15 **A** = True **B** = True **C** = True **D** = False **E** = True

Lowering the intra-ocular pressure in a patient with **normal tension glaucoma** does appear to be of some benefit. However, the pressure needs to be low enough – at least < 16 mmHg if not lower. If field loss progresses the pressure should probably be lower still; however, other factors may be important. Nocturnal hypotension may impair the optic nerve head circulation. To confirm this, 24-hour ambulatory blood pressure measurement may be necessary and a patient on systemic antihypertensive medication should have this reviewed. Other vascular factors may be important, for example vasospasm in migraine or in patients with Raynaud's phenomena. Non-compliance with topical medication is also common. Pressure spikes may be occurring and so phasing may be useful to diagnose this as increased treatment will be needed. Steroids by any route of administration can cause an intra-ocular pressure rise and should not be overlooked.

16 **A** = False **B** = True **C** = False **D** = True **E** = True

The superior and inferior temporal nerve fibres are the most vulnerable to glaucomatous damage; hence, notching occurs most commonly at these sites. Other signs suggestive of **glaucomatous optic nerve damage** are: generalized enlargement of the optic cup, especially if this is asymmetrical and progressive; vertical enlargement of the cup; loss of disc rim; splinter haemorrhages; regional pallor; exposed lamina cribosa; nasal displacement of vessels; and baring of circumlinear vessels. Peripapillary atrophy can occur in normals and in myopia.

However, it is associated with glaucoma and is sometimes considered an indication for treatment of ocular hypertension. Optic disc cupping is reversible in certain cases, for example when the intra-ocular pressure is lowered in congenital glaucoma.

17   **A** = True   **B** = False   **C** = True   **D** = False   **E** = True

Pseudoexfoliative material is widely dispersed, including the pupil margin, lens capsule, corneal endothelium and anterior hyaloid face. It has also been identified in extra-ocular sites such as the liver. Iris transillumination occurs especially at the margin of the pupil rather than at the iris periphery as in pigment dispersion syndrome. Phacodonesis is pathological mobility of the lens as a result of zonular weakness. This can make cataract surgery hazardous. Lens extraction does not reduce the production of pseudoexfoliative material. Patients present most commonly in the seventh decade.

18   **A** = True   **B** = True   **C** = False   **D** = True   **E** = True

Open-angle glaucoma occurs as a result of a

- **pretrabecular problem**, in which material enters the angle and blocks it
- **trabecular problem**, e.g. trabeculitis
- **post-trabecular problem**, e.g. raised episcleral pressure.

Angle-closure glaucoma occurs as a result of

- **pupil block**, e.g. by a large lens or posterior synechiae
- **the angle itself being closed**, e.g. because of peripheral anterior synechiae (PAS)
- the **iris root being pushed forward from behind**, e.g. by choroid effusions.

Iris neovascularization has three stages
    1. present without causing glaucoma
    2. secondary open-angle glaucoma
    3. secondary angle closure as a result of PAS.

Phacomorphic glaucoma is due to an enlarged cataractous lens causing pupil block. The Posner–Schlossman syndrome is associated with spikes of high pressure occurring with evidence of anterior chamber inflammation. Uveitis can cause PAS and so angle closure without pupil block. It can also cause pupil block by causing 360° posterior synechiae. A carotico-cavernous fistula causes open-angle glaucoma by causing a raised episcleral pressure. Angle-closure glaucoma can occur rarely as a result of choroidal effusions.

Paper 1 Answers

19 A = True B = True C = True D = True E = True

In relation to size of tumour, mortality at 5 years after enucleation is

- **small**, basal diameter up to 10 mm and less than 3 mm thick (16%)
- **medium**, 10.1–15 mm diameter and 3.1–8 mm thick (32%)
- **large**, 15 mm diameter and > 8 mm thick (53%).

Risk factors for metastatic death with **choroidal melanoma** are

- increased age at enucleation
- number of epithelioid cells per high-powered field
- nucleolar area
- closed vascular loops within the tumour
- lymphocytic infiltration
- extra-ocular extension
- rapid regression after radiotherapy
- annular extension into anterior chamber angle.

With local resection

- < 2 risk factors results in a 90% 5-year survival
- > 3 risk factors results in a 30% 4-year survival.

Adjuvant chemotherapy and immunotherapy may be of benefit to the high-risk group in the future.

20 A = False B = True C = True D = True E = False

Choroidal naevi are found in 1–6.5% of the normal population. Around 1 per 5000 per year probably progress to melanomas. Risk factors for progression are: the presence of lipofuscin, subretinal fluid, visual symptoms and a thickness of greater than 2 mm on ultrasound measurement. 'Reassuring' features are surface drusen and retinal pigment epithelial clumping.

Naevi with a thickness greater than 2 mm, subretinal fluid or lipofuscin on their surface should be followed up. If all three of these features are present then treatment is probably indicated. In the absence of any of these features follow-up is probably unnecessary.

21 A = False B = True C = True D = True E = True

The value of **investigations in anterior uveitis** is often questioned. However, some tests may be helpful, especially if appropriately directed. A raised ACE suggests a diagnosis of sarcoidosis, as does a raised calcium. Behçet's is a clinical diagnosis but can be associated with HLA B5. *Toxoplasma* serology can be useful in excluding toxoplasmosis if negative. A positive test is too common in the population to be diagnostic; however, a rising titre may indicate active infection. HLA B27 is associated with Reiter's syndrome, psoriasis, ankylosing spondylitis, ulcerative colitis and with anterior uveitis alone. A test for syphilis (e.g. VDRL) is rarely positive in anterior uveitis; however, it is one of the few causes of iritis that can be treated.

22   **A** = False   **B** = True   **C** = True   **D** = True   **E** = False

Pars planitis typically occurs in a child or young adult. Approximately 80% will develop bilateral disease. The main causes of visual loss are floaters, cystoid macular oedema, cataract and tractional retinal detachment.

23   **A** = True   **B** = False   **C** = True   **D** = True   **E** = True

Complications of **branch retinal vein occlusion** (BRVO) include:

- early
    macular oedema
    macular haemorrhage
    macular ischaemia
- late
    macular oedema, haemorrhage, ischaemia and exudates
    retinal neovascularization
    vitreous haemorrhage
    epiretinal membrane.

Isolated BRVO only very rarely induces the degree of ischaemia required to produce iris neovascularization. This is more a feature of ischaemic central retinal vein occlusions (CRVOs) and hemi-CRVOs.

24   **A** = True   **B** = True   **C** = False   **D** = True   **E** = True

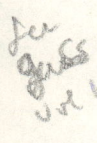

Prolonged **hypertension** (and increasing age) result in atherosclerotic vascular changes. Acutely elevated blood pressure, however, causes 'hypertensive' changes in the choroid and retina. This is typically graded as

- **grade 1**, mild generalized arteriolar constriction
- **grade 2**, focal arteriolar narrowing
- **grade 3**, as above plus retinal haemorrhages, lipid exudate, oedema and cotton wool spots
- **grade 4**, as above plus optic disc swelling.

The underlying pathology involves focal and generalized vasoconstriction with thickening of the arterial walls and endothelial cell hyperplasia. Micro- and macro-aneurysms may be found, and breakdown of the blood retinal barrier leads to exudates and oedema. Elschnig's spots are signs of focal choroidal infarction.

A 'bull's-eye' macular appearance may be found in chloroquine toxicity and cone dystrophies.

25   **A** = False **B** = True **C** = False **D** = True **E** = False

Diabetic maculopathy
The **ETDRS** recommended treatment for the following

- hard exudate within 500 µm of the fovea if associated with retinal thickening
- retinal thickening within 500 µm of the fovea
- retinal thickening greater than or equal to one disc area any part of which is within 1 disc diameter of the fovea.

Retinal thickening is synonymous with retinal oedema.

Microaneurysms alone are not an indication for treatment and neither is retinal oedema simply within the temporal arcades. Enlargement of the foveal avascular zone implies foveal ischaemia, which is not amenable to laser treatment.

26   **A** = True **B** = True **C** = True **D** = True **E** = True

Diabetic retinopathy
IRMAs reflect retinal ischaemia and are a sign of preproliferative retinopathy. The DCCT (Diabetic Control and Complications Trial) showed that the introduction of tight blood sugar control made retinopathy worsen in the first year, but following this there was a reduction in onset and progression of retinopathy and renal disease. Rapid normalization of blood sugar levels frequently worsens retinopathy. Postulated mechanisms for this phenomenon are either a reduction in retinal perfusion or an increase in growth factors such as IGF-1.

Proteinuria is found in diabetic renal disease and is a marker of microangiopathy. Treatment with ACE inhibitors appears to improve the course of nephropathy and retinopathy.

27   **A** = True **B** = True **C** = False **D** = True **E** = True

Sickle cell retinopathy results from occlusion of arterioles and venules as a result of increased blood viscosity. Occlusions are usually equatorial; however, macular vessels may also be affected. Subretinal neovascularization may occur, especially in those patients who have associated angioid streaks. Retinal ischaemia results typically in 'sea-fan' equatorial neovascularization with possible subsequent vitreous haemorrhage, tractional and rhegmatogenous retinal detachment. Ischaemic optic neuropathy is not associated.

28 **A** = True **B** = False **C** = False **D** = False **E** = False

Punctate inner choroidopathy (PIC) occurs most commonly in young myopic women. The classic fundal appearance is of a few small, white, punched out, choroidal lesions in the posterior pole. The patient is at risk of choroidal neovascularization. This may benefit from laser treatment or surgical removal. There is no vitritis and the blind spot is not enlarged. Presumed ocular histoplasmosis syndrome (POHS) has similar features to PIC but is now diagnosed only in America as histoplasmosis is not found in Europe.

Multifocal choroiditis (MIC) is associated with vitritis and more extensive choroidal lesions.

29 **A** = True **B** = True **C** = True **D** = False **E** = False

Retinitis pigmentosa-like pigmentation
Other causes include an ophthalmic artery occlusion, previous ocular trauma, calcium oxalate retinopathy and rubella retinopathy.

30 **A** = False **B** = True **C** = True **D** = False **E** = False

An ischaemic **CRVO** should be considered for prophylactic pan-retinal photocoagulation (PRP) to prevent neovascular glaucoma. An alternative is close observation and PRP at the first sign of iris neovascularization. Neovascularization at the posterior pole is far less common than in the anterior segment. It may arise after PRP for iris new vessels. Macular grid laser is not effective in treating macular oedema after CRVO. A hemi-central retinal vein occlusion has similar aetiological risk factors to a central retinal vein occlusion.

31 **A** = True **B** = False **C** = False **D** = True **E** = True

With **retinal vascular occlusions**, especially if multiple or occurring at a young age, clotting abnormalities need to be considered. A thrombophilia screen should be requested. Activated protein C resistance, or factor V Leiden, is the commonest abnormality found. A history of spontaneous abortions is suggestive of the antiphospholipid syndrome. Haemoglobin electrophoresis may detect other abnormalities, e.g. sickle cell disease in the right ethnic group. Christmas disease gives an increased risk of bleeding.

32 **A** = False **B** = True **C** = True **D** = True **E** = False

The inheritance of **Best's** is autosomal dominant with variable penetrance and expressivity, so 50% of siblings inherit the risk of developing macular dystrophy but the severity of the disease is very variable. In the early stages the fundal appearance is normal but the EOG is abnormal. The lesions can be bilateral, unilateral, multiple or single, at the macula or eccentric. The onset is usually within the first and second decade of life but the disease can begin in neonates. The visual acuity is only moderately affected until the late stages so nystagmus is not a feature.

33 **A** = True **B** = False **C** = False **D** = False **E** = True

Plain X-rays are useful in the detection of **intra-ocular foreign bodies (IOFBs)**, whereas CT scan is useful in localization and in the detection of less radio-opaque FBs. MRI is contraindicated because of the risk of displacement of ferromagnetic FBs during scanning.

When IOFBs are embedded in the retina a magnet at the pars plana should not be used as twisting and moving of the FB may cause further retinal damage. Such cases require pars plana vitrectomy and removal of the FB either with forceps or internal small rare-earth magnet.

Posterior segment perforations and scleral rupture classically cause deepening of the anterior chamber if loss of ocular contents occurs posteriorly.

Bacillus cereus causes 25% of post-traumatic endophthalmitis and typically results in fulminant infections with severe visual loss and risk of loss of the eye.

34 **A** = False **B** = True **C** = False **D** = True **E** = False

Some degree of **proliferative vitreoretinopathy** (PVR) occurs in 10% of rhegmatogenous RDs.
   Signs include:

- vitreous haze
- rolled edges of retinal breaks
- retinal wrinkling and later star folds
- retinal rigidity
- vascular tortuosity
- subretinal bands.

Predisposing factors are

- previous RD surgery
- excessive cryotherapy
- longstanding RD
- large retinal breaks
- vitreous loss at cataract surgery.

35   **A** = True   **B** = True   **C** = False   **D** = True   **E** = True

Exudative retinal detachment
Other causes include hypothyroidism, choroidal tumours and severe hypertension.

36   **A** = True   **B** = False   **C** = False   **D** = False   **E** = True

Assessment of strabismus
On cover testing in congenital esotropia the covered eye may drift upwards as well as inwards, indicating DVD. In the prism cover test the prism should point in the direction of the abnormally positioned eye. To assess fully an esotropia with a cover test an accommodative target is required, a light used as a target will not induce any accommodation. A child with a congenital esotropia may not move his eyes laterally on pursuit because of cross-fixation. When one eye is covered the uncovered eye will move laterally, which enables differentiation from bilateral VI nerve palsies.

37   **A** = False   **B** = True   **C** = False   **D** = False   **E** = False

A **microtropia** is a squint of < 10 dioptre with some degree of binocular single vision. No movement is seen on a 4-dioptre prism cover test because of a foveal suppression scotoma. It is usually associated with anisometropia and frequently causes amblyopia. Surgery is not required. It is usually an esotropia. DVD occurs in congenital esotropia.

38   **A** = True   **B** = False   **C** = True   **D** = True   **E** = False

One reason for adopting an **abnormal head posture** (AHP) is to position the eyes in the best field of binocular single vision. By being chin down the eyes are effectively elevated. With an A exotropia this decreases the size of the exotropia. An A esotropia will be worse with the chin down. Downbeat nystagmus is reduced with the eyes elevated. In paralytic squint the AHP is usually in the direction of action of the paralysed muscle. In IV nerve palsies the ability to depress the eyes is reduced

Paper 1 *Answers*

so a compensatory chin-down posture is adopted. Internuclear ophthalmoplegia is unlikely to lead to an abnormal head posture, but there can be vertical nystagmus on elevation of the eyes.

39   A = True   B = False   C = True   D = True   E = True

Delayed visual maturation (DVM) occurs when a baby shows visual responses not consistent with his chronological or developmental age in the absence of disease of the visual pathways or brain. DVM is either an isolated finding, associated with systemic disease or mental retardation, or associated with ocular disease.

The isolated form of DVM has the best visual prognosis and that associated with mental retardation the worst. The diagnosis is often retrospective as improvement often occurs before the first clinic visit.

40   A = False   B = True   C = True   D = False   E = False

Maternal **rubella** infection in the first trimester results in greater severity of prevalence of features of congenital rubella syndrome and may result in fetal death. Systemic features are neonatal rash, hepatosplenomegaly, thrombocytopenic purpura, microcephaly, osteopathy, lymphadenopathy and diabetes. Pigmentary retinopathy is found in 40%, cataracts in 20% and glaucoma in 10%. The ERG shows minimal changes in contrast to the retinal dystrophies associated with deafness.

41   A = False   B = False   C = False   D = False   E = True

The most common presenting signs of a **retinoblastoma** are leucocoria and strabismus. Other presenting features include poor vision, glaucoma, unilateral mydriasis, heterochromia, hyphaema and orbital cellulitis.

The differential diagnosis includes:

- **hereditary conditions,** such as Norrie's disease, Warburg syndrome, familial exudative vitreoretinopathy, retinal dysplasia
- **developmental anomalies** (which may cause microphthalmia), such as persistent hyperplastic primary vitreous, congenital retinal folds
- **inflammatory conditions,** such as toxocariasis (does not calcify, retinoblastoma does), metastatic endophthalmitis
- **other tumours,** such as choroidal haemangioma, astrocytic hamartoma
- **other conditions,** such as retinopathy of prematurity (low birth weight), retinal detachment.

A germinal mutation and hence the potential to be hereditary is expected if there is a family history of retinoblastoma or if it is bilateral. However, about 15% of unilateral cases have a germinal mutation. Only 6–10% of hereditary cases have a positive family history. The inheritance is autosomal dominant with a high penetrance. With a carrier mother there is a 50% chance of the sibling having the genetic potential for a retinoblastoma. Forty-five per cent will actually develop one.

42   **A** = False   **B** = False   **C** = False   **D** = True   **E** = True

The ESR is 'normal' in arteritic **AION** in 10%. Visual loss is usually more severe in arteritic disease.

Non-arteritic AION results from microvascular occlusion rather than embolism and is not associated with carotid atheroma. Patients have only a slightly increased incidence of cardiovascular disease and, unlike in central retinal artery occlusion, there is no significant shortening of life expectancy. Optic disc 'crowding' may be a factor in non-arteritic AION as many affected patients have a very low cup to disc ratio.

43   **A** = True   **B** = False   **C** = True   **D** = True   **E** = True

Benign intracranial hypertension (BIH) (or idiopathic intracranial hypertension) is a diagnosis of exclusion. A VI nerve palsy is a non-localizing sign and can simply occur as a result of raised intracranial pressure. Other neurological signs suggest another diagnosis. Raised CSF protein or cells suggest an inflammatory cause such as chronic meningitis or lupus arteritis. Long-term steroids or steroid withdrawal are associated. Steroids can be used in treatment but tend to cause weight gain and fluid retention. As weight loss is a good treatment in itself further weight gain is best avoided. The blind spots may be enlarged and the visual fields constricted. Transient obscurations of vision are associated with raised intracranial pressure, and are one of the indications for more treatment. The need for treatment is mainly based on an assessment of optic nerve function. Treatment options include weight loss, diuretics, lumbar peritoneal shunts and optic nerve sheath fenestration.

44   **A** = True   **B** = True   **C** = True   **D** = True   **E** = True

Carotid artery disease
An atherosclerotic plaque in the common carotid artery can cause a cholesterol embolus. Stenosis of the artery can lead to an ocular ischaemic syndrome, including iris neovascularization. Photopsia can also occur as a result of transient ischaemia. Choroidal detachments can occur with carotico-cavernous fistula. Horner's syndrome can occur with carotid artery dissection in the neck. Neck pain and often a history of trauma are clues to this diagnosis.

45 **A** = True   **B** = True   **C** = True   **D** = False   **E** = True

Cranial nerve palsy
Whereas a painful III nerve palsy is classically due to a posterior communicating artery aneurysm, diabetes can also cause a III nerve palsy associated with headache. The pupil is usually dilated with a III nerve palsy associated with an aneurysm and not one associated with diabetes, but not always. If there is any doubt, imaging should be performed: either carotid angiography or magnetic resonance angiography. Lid elevation on downgaze (pseudo-von Graefe sign) or on adduction occurs with aberrant regeneration of the III nerve; so does pupil miosis on adduction (pseudo-Argyll Robertson pupil). Aberrant regeneration occurs 8–12 weeks after trauma, aneurysmal compression or a tumour affecting the III nerve. It does not occur with diabetic or hypertensive neuropathy. Primary aberrant regeneration is nearly always due to a cavernous sinus meningioma.

IV nerve palsies can be congenital or acquired. Acquired cases are most commonly due to trauma or diabetes.

46 **A** = False   **B** = False   **C** = True   **D** = True   **E** = False

Optic neuritis
Colour vision is often severely reduced in relation to visual acuity. Visual evoked potential (VEP) shows a prolonged P100. The finding of a delay in the VEP in the other, apparently unaffected, eye is very suggestive of a diagnosis of multiple sclerosis. Multiple sclerosis is diagnosed by finding two or more demyelinating episodes separated by time. MRI can show areas of demyelination that may not be apparent clinically and so can help make a diagnosis of multiple sclerosis. The optic neuritis treatment trial showed that in patients with optic neuritis and four or more lesions on MRI, pulsed i.v. methylprednisolone could delay the onset of multiple sclerosis by 2 years. Using oral prednisolone alone seemed to lead to a higher recurrence rate of optic neuritis compared with no treatment at all.

47 **A** = True   **B** = False   **C** = True   **D** = True   **E** = False

In pseudopapilloedema

- the central cup is often absent, whereas spontaneous venous pulsation is preserved
- the retinal vessels frequently have an abnormal branching pattern
- there are no retinal haemorrhages, exudates, cotton wool spots or telangiectatic disc vessels
- the disc margin is irregular with abnormal peripapillary retinal pigment epithelium (RPE)
- retinal folds are not present
- there is no fluorescein leakage from disc vessels.

48   **A** = True   **B** = False   **C** = True   **D** = False   **E** = True

NF1 has dominant inheritance with incomplete penetrance. The gene defect is on chromosome 17. It is associated with the formation of multiple tumour types including neurofibromas, optic gliomas, astrocytomas and phaeochromocytomas.
   The **diagnostic criteria** are two or more of the following

- two or more Lisch nodules
- six or more *café-au-lait* patches with a diameter of at least 5 mm in prepubertal and 15 mm in post-pubertal individuals
- optic nerve glioma
- intertriginous freckling
- distinctive bony lesions (e.g. sphenoid bone dysplasia or thinning of long bone cortex)
- first-degree relative with diagnosis of NF1.

Acoustic neuroma and posterior subcapsular cataract are features of NF2.

49   **A** = False   **B** = False   **C** = True   **D** = True   **E** = True

Anisocoria
Varying the level of illumination helps to identify the affected eye. Increased anisocoria in bright light implies a failure of constriction of the larger pupil, and increased anisocoria in dim light indicates failure of dilatation of the small pupil.
   Vermiform movements may be seen in Adie's pupils, which ultimately tend to become miosed.
   Physiological anisocoria is found in 20% of the population, but generally does not exceed 1 mm.
   Botulinum toxin may cause anisocoria if absorbed into the eye. Always think of possible pharmacological causes when seeing patients with anisocoria.

50   **A** = True   **B** = True   **C** = True   **D** = True   **E** = True

Optic atrophy results from any cause of extensive ganglion cell loss.
   Causes include:

- **inherited**
   Leber's congenital amaurosis
   congenital optic atrophy
   Leber's optic atrophy
   dominant optic atrophy
- **vascular**
   ischaemic optic neuropathy
   post CRVO or central retinal artery occlusion (CRAO)

- **glaucoma**
- **metabolic**
    tobacco/alcohol amplyopia
    vitamin B12 deficiency
- **drugs**
    ethambutol
- **inflammation**
    optic neuritis
- **compression**
    sphenoid sinus mucocele
- **neoplastic**
    pituitary adenoma
    meningioma
    glioma
- **infective**
    syphilis
- **radiation neuropathy.**

51 **A** = True   **B** = True   **C** = False   **D** = False   **E** = True

CMV is a major cause of visual loss in **AIDS**. Typical findings are white retinal lesions with later haemorrhages, exudates, vascular sheathing, choroiditis and possible exudative retinal detachment. CMV may also cause optic neuritis (usually acute and anterior) and encephalitis with a wide range of manifestations.

HIV infection alone may cause early or late neurological effects. Five to ten per cent of newly infected patients develop aseptic meningitis or meningoencephalitis, and sometimes cranial nerve palsies. Long-term HIV infection may lead to HIV encephalopathy or AIDS dementia complex with global encephalitic changes. HIV may also result in retinal haemorrhages, cottonwool spots and retinal vasculitis.

CNS toxoplasmosis occurs in one-third of AIDS patients but ocular involvement is rare in the absence of pre-existing congenital choroidal toxoplasmosis scars.

Herpes simplex (HSV) and zoster (HZ) typically result in peripheral retinal necrosis, causing symptoms of floaters, photopsia, blurred vision and ocular pain. Other common manifestations of HSV and HZ in AIDS are encephalitis and radiculitis (e.g. herpes zoster ophthalmicus).

Progressive multifocal leucoencephalopathy is a destruction of white matter oligodendrocytes caused by a papovavirus. It is found in 1–4% of patients with AIDS. Ophthalmic effects include diplopia, visual field loss and cortical blindness.

Other diseases found in AIDS that may affect the visual system include:

- CNS lymphoma (usually high grade-B cell non-Hodgkin's)
- mycobacterial infection
- syphilis
- *Pneumocystis carinii* (ocular or CNS).

52   **A** = True   **B** = True   **C** = True   **D** = True   **E** = False

Myotonic dystrophy is dominantly inherited (chromosome 19) and may be confused with chronic progressive external ophthalmoplegia. The severity is often worsened in successive generations.

Features include:

- **ocular**
    ptosis
    ophthalmoplegia
    polychromatic cataracts
    miotic pupils
    near-light dissociation of pupil reactions
    pigmentary retinopathy
- **systemic**
    temporalis/masseter wasting
    frontal balding
    myopathic facies
    insulin resistance
    deafness
    cardiomyopathy
    cardiac conduction defects
    uterine atony
    testicular atrophy.

Changes begin in adolescence and the myotonia may be worsened by cold, fatigue or excitement. A characteristic feature is difficulty in relaxing the grip after a handshake. Electromyography is diagnostic.

53   **A** = True   **B** = True   **C** = True   **D** = False   **E** = False

Dorsal midbrain (Parinaud's) syndrome has the following features:

- impaired upgaze
- eyelid retraction (Collier's sign)
- convergence–retraction nystagmus (best shown with downwards rotating OKN drum)
- impaired accommodation
- near-light dissociation (constriction to near but not to light).

This syndrome results from pathology in the rostral midbrain.
Causes include:

- cerebrovascular accident (posterior cerebral artery territory)
- basilar tip pathology (e.g. aneurysm, embolus, surgical trauma)

Paper 1 *Answers*

- tumour
    - pinealoma
    - teratoma
    - germ cell tumours
- demyelination
- trauma
- neurosyphilis.

54   **A** = False   **B** = True   **C** = True   **D** = False   **E** = False

CT scan
- **advantages**
    possible with ferromagnetic materials present
    good definition of bony structures for evaluation of anatomy, fractures and bony erosion
    faster acquisition time
    cheaper than MRI
- **disadvantages**
    radiation exposure (1–2 rads for CT scan of head/orbits, 50 mrads for chest X-ray)
    reformatting images in other planes results in image degradation ('spiral CT' partially addresses this problem)
    soft tissue definition not as good as MRI
    artefact from dental amalgam and dense bone.

MRI
- **advantages**
    can display images in any plane without repositioning the patient or degrading images
    no artefact from skull base or other bony structures
    better definition of soft tissues
    flow void indicates blood flow within vessels
    no radiation exposure
- **disadvantages**
    contraindicated in the presence of ferro-magnetic metals
    no image from calcium or bone
    spatial resolution worse than CT
    takes longer than CT (so more problem with motion artefact)
    difficult for patients with claustrophobia
    problems with scanning under anaesthesia.

55   **A** = False   **B** = True   **C** = True   **D** = False   **E** = False

The **argon laser** is a gas laser producing peak emission at 488 nm (blue) and 514 nm (green) wavelengths. Argon 'green' is used in the macular area as the xanthophyll pigment of the superficial layers strongly absorbs the blue wavelength. Photocoagulation is the mode of action and tissue temperatures are raised to 80°C at the centre of a normal burn. Uses of the argon laser include pan-retinal photocoagulation for retinal ischaemia, focal and grid macular treatments, iridotomy, laser trabeculoplasty, coagulation of subretinal neovascular membranes and suture lysis. Cycloablation is performed with cryotherapy, NdYAG laser on continuous wave setting or diode laser.

56   **A** = False   **B** = False   **C** = True   **D** = True   **E** = True

Drug toxicity
Tamoxifen can cause crystalline deposits at the macular, as can canthaxanthine (a drug taken to simulate a suntan). Thioridazine causes retinal pigmentation. Toxic levels of digoxin may cause xanthopsia, a 'yellowing' of the vision. Desferrioxamine can cause a peripheral neuropathy as well as optic neuropathy.

57   **A** = True   **B** = True   **C** = False   **D** = True   **E** = True

Ocular features of **albinism** include poor vision, sensory nystagmus, strabismus, iris transillumination, foveal hypoplasia and abnormal decussation at the chiasm with up to 90% of fibres decussating.

Two rare subgroups of albinism have potentially fatal systemic abnormalities. In Chediak–Higashi syndrome oculocutaneous albinism is associated with extreme susceptibility to infection. In Hermanski–Pudlak syndrome a platelet defect causes easy bruising and bleeding.

58   **A** = True   **B** = True   **C** = False   **D** = False   **E** = False

Herpes viruses and the eye
With the advent of polymerase chain reaction (PCR) tests it is now more possible to look for viral causes of inflammatory eye diseases. The herpes family includes simplex, zoster and cytomegalovirus (CMV). Acute retinal necrosis (ARN) usually starts in peripheral retina and is associated with retinal arteritis. It can occur in a non-immunocompromised patient. Progressive outer retinal necrosis (PORN) has only been reported in AIDS patients.

59   **A** = False   **B** = True   **C** = True   **D** = False   **E** = False

Three main types of **giant cell** occur. **Foreign body** giant cells have randomly placed nuclei or nuclei at the edge of the cytoplasm; **Langerhans** type have a very peripheral pattern of nuclei (typical of tuberculosis or leprosy); **Touton's** giant cells are smaller and the nuclei are arranged in a ring at the centre of the cell. These occur in xanthogranuloma.

60   **A** = True   **B** = True   **C** = True   **D** = False   **E** = False

Ciliary body tumours
Medulloepitheliomata arise in the ciliary epithelium and usually present in childhood. Malignant medulloepitheliomata occur in adults and on histology may contain 'rosettes' resembling the Flexner–Wintersteiner rosettes of retinoblastomas. Adenomas occur in adults and can cause reduced vision as a result of contact with the lens. Adenocarcinomas are very rare malignant ciliary body tumours found in adults. Any of the tissue types of the ciliary body may cause benign or malignant tumours (although many are vanishingly rare).

Paper 2

Answers

61 **A** = False **B** = True **C** = True **D** = False **E** = False

A congenital **ptosis** is characterized by an absent or reduced skin crease of normal position with reduced levator function. An aponeurotic defect is characterized by a raised skin crease but good levator function. The ptosis of Horner's syndrome is only 2 mm. Question **C** is describing Cogan's lid twitch sign characteristic of ocular myasthenia gravis. Question **E** is describing Marcus–Gunn jaw winking. Aberrant regeneration of the III nerve can cause abnormal movement of the lid, in particular lid elevation on adduction and on downgaze.

62 **A** = False **B** = True **C** = False **D** = True **E** = True

Nasolacrimal disorders
Drainage of dacryocystitis through the skin should be avoided if possible as a fistula may form.

Congenital nasolacrimal duct obstruction frequently resolves spontaneously by the age of 1 year and syringing should be delayed until this time.

A dacryocystorhinostomy (DCR) anastomoses the lacrimal sac to the nose, so bypassing the nasolacrimal duct. Therefore, this will cure nasolacrimal duct obstruction. An external or endonasal approach can be used. Obstruction of the common canaliculus at the site of entry to the lacrimal sac can be treated with a DCR and intubation. Mid-canalicular to distal blockage may be treated with a CDCR (canalicular DCR), but more proximal blockage requires insertion of Lester Jones tubes directly from the inferior conjunctival sac into the nose.

63 **A** = False **B** = False **C** = True **D** = True **E** = True

The majority of patients with **dysthyroid eye disease** have mild ocular problems and require supportive measures such as artificial tears. Exposure keratopathy may reduce the vision and requires intensive lubrication and sometimes tarsorrhaphy.

Reduced colour vision, along with reduced acuity, relative afferent pupil defect and visual field constriction, imply optic nerve compromise. This requires urgent measures to restore vision. High-dose systemic steroids may temporarily decompress the orbit until radiotherapy or decompressive surgery is carried out.

The inferior and medial recti are most commonly involved followed by the superior and lateral recti.

Rehabilitative surgery for squint and lid retraction should only be carried out when the orbitopathy is inactive. The eyes should be aligned first followed by lid surgery if necessary.

64   **A** = True   **B** = False   **C** = True   **D** = True   **E** = False

Capillary haemangiomas (strawberry naevi) frequently appear within the first week of life, enlarge throughout the first year and 75% involute spontaneously within 4 years. They are often associated with haemangiomas on other parts of the body. There is no inheritance pattern. Large lesions may be associated with thrombocytopenia (Kossabach–Merritt syndrome). Amblyopia may develop as a result of induced astigmatism or occlusion of the visual axis. If vision is threatened intralesional triamcinolone injections may induce regression. Reported side-effects include necrosis of the skin overlying the lesion, subcutaneous fat atrophy and embolic visual loss. Surgery is generally only suitable for small lesions because of the difficulty of haemostasis. Other reported treatment modalities include systemic steroids, systemic interferon alpha and radiotherapy.

Facial 'port wine stain' (naevus flammeous) in Sturge–Weber syndrome is associated with glaucoma.

65   **A** = True   **B** = False   **C** = True   **D** = False   **E** = False

About 50% of **lacrimal gland enlargements** are due to inflammatory or lymphoproliferative processes. The other 50% are half due to benign mixed cell tumours and half-carcinomas. Inflammatory processes include infective dacroadenitis, sarcoidosis, Wegener's granulomatosis, pseudotumour and lymphomas. ANCA is a test for Wegener's granulomatosis. A benign tumour should not be biopsied but removed en bloc via a lateral orbitotomy. A suspected malignant tumour should be biopsied and, as the prognosis is poor palliative, radiotherapy may be a better option than exenteration. If a benign tumour is inadvertently biopsied then the rest of the gland should be removed with the biopsy tract and overlying skin because of the risk of seeding tumour cells.

66   **A** = True   **B** = True   **C** = True   **D** = False   **E** = True

Conjunctival cicatrization may occur after acute injury with subsequent scarring or be slowly progressive.

Causes include:

- **physical**, radiotherapy, alkali burn
- **infection**, trachoma, membranous conjunctivitis
- **oculocutaneous**, ocular cicatricial pemphigoid, Stevens–Johnson syndrome, linear IgA disease
- **systemic disease**, graft versus-host disease, paraneoplastic syndromes
- **drugs**, practolol, topical drops (e.g. pilocarpine).

67   **A** = False   **B** = False   **C** = True   **D** = True   **E** = True

Vernal keratoconjunctivitis, adult atopic keratoconjunctivitis and giant papillary conjunctivitis (GPC) are all characterized by a papillary conjunctival response.

GPC, unlike the other two, is probably not a true allergic response but is related to chronic irritation as a result of contact lens wear, ocular prostheses and sutures on the ocular surface.

Vernal is a seasonal condition commonest in boys with a history of allergy. Elevated IgE levels in tears and serum, and an eosinophilia, may be found. Symptoms include itching, redness, watering and mucus discharge. Signs include giant papillae on the upper tarsal conjunctiva with stringy mucus discharge, limbal papillary swellings, which may develop white central dots (Tranta's dots), and keratopathy. The keratopathy consists of epithelial opacities and punctate staining, macroerosions, subepithelial scarring and arcus lipoides. Changes are usually most marked in the upper cornea.

Adult atopic keratoconjunctivitis is a more severe and visually threatening condition that is not generally seasonal. It is found in association with eczema and other allergic conditions.

Keratoconus is associated with atopy and may be related to excessive eye rubbing.

68   **A** = True   **B** = True   **C** = False   **D** = False   **E** = True

Astigmatism is one of the main problems of **corneal grafting**. Using a donor button slightly larger than the host trephine tends to decrease the level of astigmatism. Large grafts are more likely to reject because of proximity of the donor tissue to the host vasculature, whereas small grafts tend to have more astigmatism. The benefit of HLA matching is not proved and is not routinely carried out.

Adverse factors for grafting include: a poor ocular environment, e.g. lid disease or dry eyes; active corneal disease; corneal vascularization; ocular disease such as untreated glaucoma or uveitis. Some disease processes may recur such as herpes simplex and corneal dystrophies.

Paper 2 *Answers*

69   **A** = False   **B** = False   **C** = True   **D** = True   **E** = False

Eyes with **chemical injuries** should be irrigated immediately (except when caused by CS gas, when blowing warm air is recommended) and before detailed assessment is performed. The lids should be double-everted when particulate chemicals such as lime are involved. Topical steroids are used in the first week to 10 days to reduce the damage caused by inflammation. Following this, in the presence of a persistent epithelial defect, they increase the risk of sterile corneal perforation. Topical ascorbic acid replaces depleted local stores and assists in collagen synthesis. Topical antibiotics are used prophylactically.

Acids may cause severe ocular injury, but in general alkalis such as ammonia and sodium hydroxide penetrate the cornea more rapidly and cause more severe damage to the anterior segment and limbus.

70   **A** = False   **B** = True   **C** = True   **D** = True   **E** = False

The differential diagnosis of **peripheral corneal ulceration** includes:

local/isolated ocular conditions

- staphylococcal hypersensitivity (commonest)
- dry eye
- exposure keratopathy
- dellen
- vernal keratoconjunctivitis
- herpes simplex or zoster keratitis
- Terrien's marginal degeneration
- Mooren's ulcer (collagen vascular disorders must be excluded)
- pellucid marginal degeneration

systemic/generalized conditions

- collagen vascular diseases
    rheumatoid arthritis
    SLE
    polyarteritis nodosa
    relapsing polychondritis
    Wegener's granulomatosis
- acne rosacea.

71   **A** = True   **B** = False   **C** = True   **D** = False   **E** = True

Corneal ulcers
The following are useful **culture media**:

- blood agar (aerobes)
- chocolate agar (*Neisseria* and *Haemophilus*)
- Sabouraud's (fungi)
- thioglycolate (facultative anaerobes)
- brain–heart infusion (fungi).

Rose-Bengal stains the cells at the edge of a viral ulcer, fluorescein stains the base.

C. diphtheriae, *N. meningitidis* and *N. gonorrhoeae* can cause an ulcer with intact corneal epithelium. Most other infections have a predisposing factor, e.g. contact lenses, dry eyes, neurotrophic keratopathy, adnexal infection, corneal disease, immunosuppression.

72   **A** = True   **B** = False   **C** = True   **D** = True   **E** = True

Keratoconus
About 5% have a family history, although no definite form of inheritance has been established. Eye rubbing is thought to be the most common association.
Other associations include:

- eye conditions
    ectopia lentis
    retinitis pigmentosa
    congenital cataract
    aniridia
    Leber's congenital amaurosis
- systemic conditions
    atopic dermatitis
    Marfan's syndrome
    Ehlers–Danlos syndrome
    osteogenesis imperfecta.

73   **A** = True   **B** = True   **C** = False   **D** = False   **E** = True

When performing **LASIK** a corneal suction ring is applied that elevates the intra-ocular pressure to 65 mmHg for a short time. A microkeratome cuts a superficial corneal flap, which is hinged nasally. Following photoablation to the exposed stromal surface, the stromal bed is irrigated and the flap replaced. No sutures are required. Pressing on the corneal periphery induces wrinkles on the flap surface if the flap is adherent. This is known as the striae test. Flaps may be elevated for retreatment with ease up to 3 months following LASIK and probably for much longer than this.

74 **A** = True **B** = False **C** = True **D** = False **E** = True

The aetiology of **acquired cataract** includes:

- **advancing age**
- **intra-ocular inflammation**
- **trauma**
    physical, blunt/penetrating
    chemical, severe alkali injury
    radiation, infra-red, glass-blowers' cataract
    gamma ray, radiotherapy
- **ocular surgery**
    vitrectomy
    trabeculectomy
- **drugs**
    corticosteroids
    anticholinesterases
    phenothiazines
- **degenerative eye disease**
    high myopia
    retinitis pigmentosa
- **systemic conditions**
    diabetes mellitus
    myotonic dystrophy
    Down's syndrome
    atopy
    Wilson's disease
    hypocalcaemia.

Amyloidosis may cause vitreous and corneal deposits but is not associated with cataract.

75 **A** = False **B** = True **C** = True **D** = False **E** = True

Cataracts in children
Anterior polar cataracts affect the lens capsule and anterior subcapsular cortex and are frequently dominantly inherited. Unless very large the vision is usually minimally affected.

Posterior polar cataracts are near the optical nodal point of the eye and so affect the vision much more profoundly.

Lamellar cataracts may be familial or represent transient toxic events during lens development.

Congenital rubella often causes white nuclear opacities or 'total' cataract. A brisk uveitis may follow cataract surgery, possibly as a result of release of viral particles.

76   A = False   B = False   C = True   D = False   E = False

Traumatic glaucoma
Glaucoma as a result of angle recession occurs in only less than 10% and then only if at least three-quarters of the angle is recessed. The IOP may be initially high but usually falls and then there may be a late rise up to 10 or more years later. Glaucoma related to angle recession should be in the differential for unilateral open-angle glaucoma.
   Ghost cell glaucoma occurs with vitreous haemorrhage in an aphakic eye.
   Secondary glaucomas frequently cause elevated intra-ocular pressure without glaucomatous nerve damage, at least initially, as the optic nerve is otherwise healthy.
   Lead is inert. Iron and copper can cause inflammation and may cause glaucoma.
   A cyclodialysis may cause a drop in intra-ocular pressure rather than a rise.

77   A = True   B = True   C = False   D = True   E = True

Gonioscopy
The Zeiss gonioscope has four mirrors. All four quadrants of the angle can be seen at once with minimal rotation, and coupling fluid is not required. The lens can be used for indentation gonioscopy to see if the angle can be opened and so is useful for looking for peripheral anterior synechiae. The trabecular meshwork becomes increasingly pigmented with age, especially in the inferior part. Pathological causes of pigmentation include pigment dispersion syndrome, blunt trauma, anterior uveitis, following acute angle-closure glaucoma, in diabetics after cataract surgery and with naevus of Ota. The abnormal vessels in the angle in Fuch's can cause bleeding, for example at cataract surgery. Other causes of abnormal angle vessels are iris neovascularization in response to ischaemia and chronic anterior uveitis.

78   A = True   B = True   C = False   D = False   E = True

Congenital glaucoma
Rieger's and Axenfeld's have autosomal dominant inheritance, unlike Peter's anomaly, which is autosomal recessive. Posterior embryotoxon is seen in 15% of the normal population but is also a feature of Axenfeld's. Primary congenital glaucoma is mainly sporadic; 10% are inherited in a recessive fashion. Haab's striae are horizontal lines in Descemet's. Trauma from forceps, for example, causes more typically vertical splits in Descemet's membrane. Plexiform neurofibromas of the upper lid occur in type 1 neurofibromatosis and are associated with glaucoma.

79 **A** = True **B** = False **C** = False **D** = True **E** = True

Glaucoma surgery
For a successful trabeculectomy it is not necessary to remove trabecular tissue. Indeed the occurrence of a hyphaema is less likely if tissue is removed anterior to the trabeculum in clear cornea.

After a trabeculectomy, the pressure can be adjusted by carrying out argon suture lysis. Nylon sutures are best used for this. Adjustable sutures can be used as an alternative to suture lysis.

A post-operative leak can be helped by padding and using Diamox to decrease aqueous production and so reducing flow through the hole. Additional measures include decreasing the dose of topical steroid temporarily, using a bandage contact lens or a Simmond's shield, or resuturing the conjunctiva and injecting fluid or viscoelastic into the anterior chamber if a paracentesis is available. It may be necessary to drain choroidal detachments if anterior chamber reformation is attempted.

80 **A** = False **B** = True **C** = True **D** = False **E** = True

There are two main cell types in **melanomas**: spindle and epithelioid. There are two subtypes of spindle cells: spindle A and spindle B. Spindle A are slender cells with elongated nuclei. Spindle B cells are plumper with more ovoid nuclei. Epithelioid cells are large round cells with eccentric round nuclei. This cell type has the worst prognosis. Most iris melanomas are spindle type and grow slowly; very rarely have they been reported to metastasize. Metastases are the commonest ocular tumours, mainly from breast and lung.

81 **A** = True **B** = False **C** = True **D** = True **E** = True

In **heterochromia** the affected iris may be lighter or darker depending on the cause. Causes include:

- **congenital**
    ocular/oculocutaneous melanocytosis
    iris hamartoma
    Horner's syndrome
    Waardenberg's syndrome (+white forelock, deafness, telecanthus)
- **acquired**
    chronic uveitis
    Fuch's cyclitis
    juvenile xanthogranuloma

iridocorneal endothelial syndrome
siderosis
intra-ocular foreign body
haemosiderosis
diffuse iris naevus
iris melanoma
retinoblastoma
posterior pole malignant melanoma
metastatic tumour/lymphoma/leukaemia.

82   **A** = True   **B** = True   **C** = True   **D** = False   **E** = True

A raised IOP often occurs with a herpes-associated **anterior uveitis**. Fibrinous uveitis is more common in diabetics and if the patient is HLA B27 positive. It is important to look for cystoid macular oedema in a patient with anterior uveitis and reduced vision. This tends to occur more commonly in a patient with anterior uveitis who is HLA B27 positive. Granulomatous uveitis is associated with 'mutton fat' or large KPs. Causes include sarcoidosis, toxoplasmosis, tuberculosis, sympathetic ophthalmia, Vogt–Koyanagi–Harada syndrome (VKH).

Anterior uveitis may be caused by a posterior focus such as toxoplasmosis.

83   **A** = False   **B** = True   **C** = True   **D** = True   **E** = True

Systemic associations of uveitis
The four major features of Behçet's syndrome are

- oral ulceration
- genital ulceration
- skin lesions, including erythema nodosum, pustules and ulceration
- uveitis.

Sarcoidosis is a multisystem disorder and may present acutely with erythema nodosum.

Reiter's syndrome comprises urethritis, conjunctivitis and seronegative arthritis. Twenty per cent may develop acute iritis.

APMPPE may be preceded by a flu-like illness and erythema nodosum.

VKH is a multisystem disorder including cutaneous (alopecia, poliosis, vitiligo) and neurological (headache, meningism, deafness) signs as well as anterior and posterior uveitis.

84   **A** = False   **B** = False   **C** = True   **D** = True   **E** = True

Angioid streaks represent breaks in Bruch's membrane.
Associations include:

- pseudoxanthoma elasticum
- Ehlers–Danlos syndrome
- optic nerve drusen
- sickle cell anaemia
- Paget's disease
- 50% are idiopathic.

On ophthalmoscopy they are dark red or brown bands radiating from the disc. Hyperfluorescence is usually seen in the early phase of angiography as a result of retinal pigment epithelial atrophy overlying the streaks, although masking of the choroidal fluorescence occasionally occurs. Choroidal neovascularization is the greatest threat to vision. In view of the risk of choroidal rupture and subsequent choroidal neovascularization with relatively minor blunt trauma, safety glasses are often recommended.

85   **A** = False   **B** = True   **C** = True   **D** = False   **E** = False

Central serous chorioretinopathy (CSCR; previously known as central serous retinopathy) is thought to be due to leakage of fluid through the RPE and possibly impaired 'pumping' function of the RPE. Viral illnesses are not associated. Symptoms include micropsia, metamorphopsia, blurred vision and impaired colour vision. Fundal changes include localized elevation of the neuroretina at the macula and pigment epithelial mottling. Pigmentary changes may be seen in the other eye. In older patients with CSCR an important differential diagnosis is exudative age-related macular degeneration with elevation of the retinal pigment epithelium. Features suggesting CSCR are an absence of subretinal blood, lipid or drusen and the small degree of leakage on fluorescein angiography (FFA) relative to the extent of subretinal fluid. However, lipid is occasionally deposited. Typical FFA findings are a small hyperfluorescent leak beginning early in the run and slowly spreading to fill the area of retinal elevation. The 'smokestack' sign is present only in 10%.

86   **A** = False   **B** = False   **C** = False   **D** = False   **E** = True

Clinically significant macular oedema, i.e. requiring treatment, as defined by the ETDRS (Early Treatment Diabetic Retinopathy Study) is: retinal thickening (oedema) with or without exudate within 500 µm of the fovea or retinal thickening greater than a disc diameter in size within one disc diameter of the fovea.

Risk of severe visual loss with moderate to severe new vessels at the disc without vitreous haemorrhage is 25% without treatment.

Two to three thousand burns are usually required for pan-retinal photocoagulation (PRP) using a 200- to 500-μm spot size. The actual spot size varies depending on the lens used. It is argued that using a 200-μm spot size provides adequate treatment and better preserves a driving visual field.

PRP may make macular oedema worse, so maculopathy should be treated before PRP if possible in patients over 40. In younger patients macular problems may resolve after PRP.

87   **A** = True   **B** = True   **C** = False   **D** = True   **E** = False

Diabetic retinopathy
In pregnancy pre-existing retinopathy may get worse, and so such patients require close follow-up. The retinopathy may settle again after delivery. Patients without retinopathy probably will not develop it if diabetic control is good.

Preproliferative changes include venous beading and dilatation, venous loops and reduplication, IRMAs, large blotch haemorrhages and cotton wool spots.

Renal disease and hypertension can make macular oedema worse.

88   **A** = True   **B** = True   **C** = False   **D** = True   **E** = True

The retinal findings in **sickle cell retinopathy** are: salmon patches (superficial haemorrhages), black sunbursts (chorioretinal scars), sea fan neovascularization. Neovascularization is more likely to self-thrombose than in diabetics but argon laser treatment may be required. Non-retinal findings are: corkscrew-shaped conjunctival vessels, ischaemic patches of iris and iris neovascularization.

89   **A** = False   **B** = True   **C** = True   **D** = False   **E** = True

Causes of **night blindness**:

- **inherited, stationary**
    congenital stationary night blindness
    fundus albipunctatus
    Oguchi disease
- **inherited, progressive**
    retinitis pigmentosa
    choroideraemia
    gyrate atrophy
    Goldman–Favre syndrome
    choroidal atrophy

- **acquired**
    vitamin A deficiency
    desferrioxamine therapy
    (pan-retinal photocoagulation).

90   A = False   B = True   C = False   D = True   E = True

Chloroquine and hydroxychloroquine
Corneal deposits are much commoner in CQ therapy than HCQ and usually disappear within 6–8 weeks of cessation of therapy. Although corneal deposits are related to tissue concentration of CQ or HCQ, they are not linked to maculopathy. There are no fundoscopic changes in early maculopathy. Electrophysiological tests, fluorescein angiography and visual acuity are also frequently normal. Early retinopathy is characterized by relative paracentral visual field defects, which are detectable by Amsler grid (especially red on black Amsler) or formal static perimetry. Early retinopathy often resolves on cessation of CQ or HCQ therapy. In established retinopathy the absolute field defects frequently progress, a bull's-eye maculopathy develops and the visual prognosis is poor. This is much rarer with HCQ therapy than CQ therapy.

91   A = True   B = False   C = False   D = True   E = True

Stargardt's macular dystrophy can also be termed atrophic macular dystrophy with flecks. If flecks occur alone this is termed fundus flavimaculatus. Stargardt's presents during the first and second decade with poor vision. Fundus flavimaculatus usually presents in adults. Such patients may later develop macular lesions. A fluorescein angiogram may show a dark choroid; this is due to masking of the normal choroidal fluorescence, not pathology in the choroid. Flecks of recent origin mask choroidal fluorescence and in the later stages of the disease they act as window defects and so cause hyperfluorescence.

The retinal blood vessels are usually normal in calibre but they may become narrowed late in the disease process. Blood vessels become narrowed in retinitis pigmentosa and in vasculitic processes. Peripheral fields and vision in the dark are normal.

92   A = True   B = True   C = True   D = True   E = False

Retinal arterial occlusions
Homocystinuria may cause arterial occlusions, especially with general anaesthesia. The heterozygote form is also associated with vascular occlusions but does not have other systemic features. Acute retinal necrosis is characterized by peripheral

retinal necrosis, panuveitis and retinal arteritis. It is caused by herpes zoster. Giant cell arteritis can cause a central retinal artery occlusion, although ischaemic optic neuropathy is the most common ocular manifestation.

93   **A** = True   **B** = True   **C** = False   **D** = True   **E** = False

Diets in ophthalmic disease
Refsum's disease causes a pigmentary retinopathy with night blindness and visual field constriction. A phytanic acid-free diet may help prevent progression. Abetalipoproteinaemia also causes a pigmentary retinopathy; vitamin E supplements may be beneficial. Progression of gyrate atrophy may be slowed by a diet low in protein and arginine, with pyridoxine (B6) supplements. Diets do not influence Stickler's syndrome or choroideraemia.

94   **A** = False   **B** = False   **C** = False   **D** = True   **E** = True

Intra-ocular foreign bodies (IOFBs) may be classified as either inert or reactive, **inert** (when sterile)

- stone
- ceramics/glass
- sand
- plastic

reactive

- (minimal/mild)
    zinc
    aluminium
- (marked/severe)
    copper
    iron.

Small zinc or aluminium IOFBs may become encapsulated and not lead to any toxicity.

Pure copper causes acute chalcosis with severe intra-ocular inflammation. Alloys with <85% copper may cause chronic chalcosis. Limiting membranes are particularly affected with Descemet's deposits (as in Wilson's disease), 'sunflower' cataracts, green iris discolouration and metallic flecks in the macular region and on retinal vessels.

Iron IOFBs result in siderosis, the severity of which depends on the size of the IOFB. Ferric ions lead to the production of oxidant radicals, which damage cell membranes and enzyme systems. Retinal photoreceptors and pigment epithelia are most commonly affected, resulting in blurred vision, night blindness and visual field constriction. Signs include corneal stromal rust coloured staining, iris heterochromia, reduced pupil reactivity, retinal pigmentary changes, optic atrophy and secondary open-angle glaucoma.

ERG is useful for detecting or monitoring retinal toxicity if any doubt exists. Removal may be indicated if the ERG deteriorates on serial testing.

95 **A** = True **B** = True **C** = False **D** = True **E** = False

Absolute indications for vitrectomy in rhegmatogenous retinal detachment are controversial; however, in general they include:

- macular breaks
- giant retinal tears
- fibrovascular or fibrocellular proliferation
- large or multiple posterior breaks
- requirement for internal search because of media opacity.

Posterior vitreous detachment is almost universally present in rhegmatogenous retinal detachment.

96 **A** = False **B** = False **C** = True **D** = True **E** = False

Retinoschisis is usually bilateral and inferotemporal with non-shifting fluid. There may be an absolute (rather than relative) visual field defect. Tobacco dust is not found in the vitreous in the absence of an outer leaf break and pigment epithelial demarcation lines are not present in retinoschisis.

Exudative detachments have a smooth surface with no corrugations or retinal breaks. Shifting fluid may be seen and a solid mass may be detected on ophthalmoscopy or B-scan ultrasound.

Choroidal detachments often occur in association with hypotony and are limited by the vortex vein exit sites. They usually have a darker appearance than neurosensory retinal detachment.

In tractional retinal detachment the detached retina is concave. There is usually a demonstrable cause such as proliferative diabetic retinopathy. Surgery is often not performed unless the macula becomes involved. Retinal breaks and subsequent rhegmatogenous detachment may occur.

97 **A** = False **B** = True **C** = False **D** = False **E** = True

Vertical squints
A positive Bielschowsky head-tilt test involves the paretic eye elevating on head tilt to the affected side because of the unopposed action of the superior rectus. Surgery

for a IV nerve palsy may involve weakening of the overacting ipsilateral antagonist, the inferior oblique or the contralateral agonist, the inferior rectus. Other procedures include superior oblique tuck or a Harada Ito type operation. Brown's syndrome causes restriction of elevation on adduction. An upshoot may occur in Duane's syndrome. Inferior oblique overaction is common with an esotropia.

98 **A** = True   **B** = True   **C** = True   **D** = True   **E** = True

Associations of Duane's syndrome
Other associations include lens opacities, microphthalmos and persistent pupillary membrane. Klippel–Feil syndrome is the fusion of cervical vertebrae. Goldenhar's syndrome is bilateral limbal dermoids, preauricular skin tags, oral fistulae, upper lid colobomas and cervical spine anomalies.

99 **A** = False   **B** = False   **C** = True   **D** = True   **E** = True

Reasons for an **abnormal head posture**
ocular

- to increase field of binocular single vision
- to increase visual acuity, e.g. by finding a null point with nystagmus, chin up with ptosis

non-ocular

- torticollis, deafness, balance problems, cervical spine problems.

In paralytic strabismus the head is moved in the direction that the non-working muscle would have moved the eye.
A left VI palsy may cause a face turn to the left. A left IV palsy may cause the head posture described in stem **B**.

100 **A** = True   **B** = True   **C** = True   **D** = False   **E** = True

The onset of **infantile esotropia** is before 6 months and is most commonly between 3 and 6 months. It is a large esotropia (> 30°). Cross-fixation is often seen and the prognosis for binocular single vision is poor. As well as the above features overaction of the inferior obliques is commonly seen.

101 **A** = False   **B** = True   **C** = False   **D** = True   **E** = False

Aniridia may result from abnormal neuroectoderm and neural crest development. Glaucoma is common, although not typically present at birth, and results from poor development of the angle, forward bowing of the ciliary processes and residual iris root, peripheral anterior synechiae and corneal endothelial ingrowth into the angle. Response to topical medications and conventional filtration surgery is often poor and tube drainage procedures are often required. Cataract is also common and may be complicated by ectopia lentis. Despite an absence of smooth muscle in the residual iris stumps, active ciliary body accommodation remains intact. Other ocular abnormalities include foveal and optic nerve hypoplasia and corneal opacification.

Sporadic cases are associated with Wilms' tumour in between a quarter and a third of patients before the age of three. A deletion at 11p13 has been shown in these cases.

102 **A** = False   **B** = False   **C** = True   **D** = False   **E** = True

Ophthalmia neonatorum is a notifiable disease. The time of onset gives some guide to the organism responsible

- within 1 day, chemical toxicity (e.g. silver nitrate drops)
- within 2–4 days, gonococcal (usually severe/purulent)
- within 1 week, other bacterial (e.g. streptococci, *Staph. aureus*, *Haemophilus* spp.)
- within 2 weeks, *Chlamydia*.

Silver nitrate drop prophylaxis is no longer routinely used in this country as the incidence of gonococcal conjunctivitis is so low. Samples should be sent for urgent Gram stain, Giemsa stain and bacterial and viral culture. Most cases (including herpes simplex) should be treated with systemic as well as topical medication because of the risk of systemic infection.

103 **A** = False   **B** = False   **C** = True   **D** = False   **E** = True

Cloudy cornea at birth
Careful examination (general anaesthesia may be required) with measurement of corneal diameter and intra-ocular pressure allows diagnosis of most causes of corneal opacity at birth. In corneal dermoid the opacity is usually found at the limbus, commonly inferotemporally. Congenital glaucoma may be unilateral or bilateral and important features are enlarged corneal diameter (> 12 mm) and elevated intra-ocular pressure. Congenital hereditary endothelial dystrophy is a bilateral condition with diffuse corneal cloudiness and increased corneal thickness. The intra-ocular pressure and corneal diameter are normal. Glaucoma is not associated with Hurler's syndrome.

Causes of cloudy cornea include

- sclerocornea
- dermoid
- forceps injury
- congenital glaucoma
- mucopolysaccharidoses/lipidoses
- congenital hereditary endothelial dystrophy
- congenital hereditary stromal dystrophy
- posterior corneal defects e.g. Peters' syndrome.

104 **A** = True   **B** = True   **C** = True   **D** = True   **E** = False

The diagnosis of **giant cell arteritis** requires a good history: Headaches and stiffness are typical but not always present, jaw claudication is pathognomonic. A high erythrocyte sedimentation rate (ESR) is usual, although not invariable. The CRP will usually be raised. As no one test is 100% sensitive and specific, a range of tests may be required to justify potential long-term steroid use. Von Willebrand factor is non-specific but is an indicator of vascular endothelial damage. A temporal artery biopsy is the most specific test; this can be positive up to 1 week after starting steroids. Two centimetres should be taken and examined with multiple sections to detect 'skip lesions'. However, a negative biopsy cannot entirely rule out the diagnosis. A normocytic normochromic anaemia may be present.

Protein electrophoresis is useful in excluding one of the differentials that could cause a high ESR, namely myeloma.

105 **A** = False   **B** = False   **C** = False   **D** = True   **E** = False

Horner's syndrome consists of a mild ptosis, elevation of the lower lid giving rise to apparent enophthalmos, and a miosed pupil that is more obvious in dim lighting. The pupil reacts normally to light and near. Decreased sweating occurs if the lesion is proximal to the superior cervical ganglion. Heterochromia may occur with Horner's that is congenital or occurring in early infancy. Adrenaline 1:1000 will dilate a post-ganglionic Horner's but not a normal pupil. Longstanding cases of Adie's pupil may have a small pupil; however, the pupil reacts slowly to light and near, and tonic sectorial vermiform movements of the pupil may be visible on the slit lamp.

106 **A** = True   **B** = False   **C** = False   **D** = True   **E** = True

Eponymous clinical phenomena
B and **C** should be swapped to give the correct names to the phenomena. **A**, **B** and

Paper 2 *Answers*   81

C all occur in multiple sclerosis. Cogan's lid twitch is seen when a patient with myasthenia is asked to look in the primary position after downgaze. The eyelid gives an upward twitch before settling into its usual position. Anton's syndrome is the denial of visual loss, which may occur in patients who are cortically blind.

107 **A** = False   **B** = True   **C** = True   **D** = True   **E** = False

Fourth nerve palsy may be congenital or acquired. In congenital palsy, review of old photographs of the patient usually shows the presence of a head tilt from an early age, and the vertical fusion range is usually increased over 3 dioptres.

Acquired palsies are most commonly traumatic and are frequently bilateral. Excyclotorsion greater than 10° suggests bilateral involvement.

Microvascular occlusion is more common in elderly patients with IV palsy.

108 **A** = True   **B** = True   **C** = False   **D** = True   **E** = False

Optic neuritis is classically associated with pain on eye movement. Central visual acuity gets worse over 2 weeks, is stable for 2 weeks and gets better over 2 weeks. If there is no visual recovery or any atypical features are present, another diagnosis should be considered. Visual acuity usually returns to normal but visual function (such as colour vision) may never fully recover.

Anterior ischaemic optic neuropathy (non-arteritic) is usually painless, associated with sudden loss of vision and an altitudinal field defect. Although some visual recovery may occur it is not the norm.

Papilloedema is nearly always bilateral, painless and usually does not affect the visual acuity, although visual obscurations may occur. If it becomes severe or chronic, visual defects may occur. These include enlargement of the blind spot, generalized field constriction and an inferior nasal defect. Colour vision and visual acuity may also be reduced.

109 **A** = False   **B** = True   **C** = True   **D** = False   **E** = True

Visual fields
Anterior ischaemic optic neuropathy typically causes an altitudinal field defect. Bilaterally increased blind spots in severe papilloedema can mimic a bitemporal hemianopia. A craniopharyngioma presses on the optic chiasm from above, so initially will cause an inferior bitemporal field defect. The more anterior a lesion is behind the chiasm the more incongruous a field defect is likely to be.

110 **A** = False   **B** = False   **C** = True   **D** = True   **E** = True

Both **neurofibromatosis** type 1 and 2 (NF1 and NF2) have autosomal dominant inheritance with variable penetrance. Fifty per cent of siblings of an affected individual will therefore have some features.

Astrocytic hamartomas are found in NF1 and also in tuberous sclerosis. Subungual fibromas are nail-bed hamartomas found in tuberous sclerosis. Brushfield spots occur on the iris in Down's syndrome.

111   **A** = False   **B** = True   **C** = True   **D** = False   **E** = True

Myasthenia gravis is a rare (4 in 100 000) autoimmune condition characterized by variable fatiguability of extra-ocular or systemic skeletal muscle. IgG anti-acetylcholine receptor antibodies are detectable in about 50% of those with ocular myasthenia and 80–95% of those with generalized myasthenia. Ninety per cent of all myasthenia patients have ocular involvement at some stage in the course of the disease, and in 75% this is the presenting complaint.

Myasthenia can mimic any type of ocular motility defect or ptosis. Variability during and between tests and fatigability are important clues to the diagnosis. The pupils are not affected.

Electromyography shows reduction in muscle fibre evoked potentials after repetitive supramaximal stimulation at 3–5 Hz. There is also a 'jitter' response on single-fibre testing.

Surgery for both ptosis and squint should be avoided in the early stages.

Medical treatment may involve anti-cholinesterase treatment, corticosteroids or immunosuppression. Thymectomy may be of benefit in resistant cases.

112   **A** = False   **B** = True   **C** = True   **D** = True   **E** = True

Recognized causes of **toxic or nutritional optic neuropathy** are

- **drugs**
    ethambutol
    rifampicin
    chloramphenicol
- **toxins**
    lead
    methanol
- **vitamin deficiency**
    thiamine (B6)
    cobalamin (B12).

113   **A** = True   **B** = False   **C** = True   **D** = True   **E** = True

Conditions worsened in pregnancy
Conditions sensitive to hormonal and cardiovascular alterations are frequently exacerbated by the physiological changes during pregnancy. Known pre-existing conditions should be monitored closely. These include:

- diabetic retinopathy
- pituitary adenoma
- meningioma
- uveal melanoma
- Graves' disease
- haemangioma.

114 **A** = True **B** = False **C** = True **D** = True **E** = False

The **mitochondrial myopathies** are inherited conditions transmitted by maternal mitochondria. Progressive weakness of the extra-ocular and sometimes facial muscles occurs. Although asymmetry may be found, diplopia is rarely a symptom. Orbicularis weakness may result in exposure keratopathy and this should be borne in mind if ptosis surgery is performed. Patients should undergo cardiac evaluation, as in Kearn–Sayre syndrome (one of the myopathies) heart block may occur. Pigmentary retinopathy and deafness may also be found. Mitochondrial analysis frequently shows DNA deletions. 'Ragged-red' fibres are seen within biopsied muscle on light microscopy with Masson trichrome staining.

115 **A** = True **B** = True **C** = True **D** = True **E** = True

Disordered visual perception
In **Charles Bonnet syndrome** visual hallucinations occur as a result of (usually recent) visual loss. The hallucinations are usually formed and commonly include faces, walking figures or animals. The patient realizes that the hallucinations are not real. The cause of visual loss may be at any point in the visual pathway. If the cause of visual loss can be cured, the syndrome may resolve, e.g. cataract surgery.

Alexia is the inability to read despite relatively normal vision. Large lesions of the left occipital lobe may produce a right hemianopia and also prevent fibres coming from the right occipital lobe to the left angular gyrus (parietal lobe). The angular gyrus of the dominant (usually left) parietal lobe is involved in reading and writing.

Patients with **visual neglect** ignore one side of visual space. This commonly occurs with right parietal lesions.

Visual agnosia is the inability to recognize objects by sight in the presence of relatively normal vision, although the ability to recognize them by other means such as touch or language is retained. Usually bilateral inferior occipital lesions are the cause.

116 **A** = True   **B** = True   **C** = True   **D** = True   **E** = True

Pan-retinal photocoagulation
Central scotoma may occur either as a result of a misplaced burn at the macula or from macular oedema induced by the PRP. Rhegmatogenous retinal detachment may result from contraction of regressing new vessels leading to retinal break formation. Studies on the effect of laser treatment on the therapist have been equivocal but it is recommended to avoid using argon blue, rather to use green.

117 **A** = True   **B** = True   **C** = True   **D** = False   **E** = False

Early neovascularization may regress with adequate PRP, so it is argued that in ischaemic CRVO prophylactic PRP may not be needed and treatment only given in those developing iris new vessels. This has the potential advantage of preserving peripheral visual field in some patients.

Neovascularization usually begins at the pupil margin. However, as neovascularization may occur only in the angle, gonioscopy should be carried out on patients considered at risk.

Iris neovascularization may result from any cause of profound posterior segment ischaemia. These include:

- diabetic retinopathy
- CRVO or CRAO
- carotid occlusive disease
- chronic uveitis
- chronic retinal detachment
- intra-ocular tumour
- retinal vascular disease (e.g. Coat's disease).

118 **A** = True   **B** = False   **C** = True   **D** = True   **E** = True

Electrodiagnostic testing
The VEP measures function from the fovea through the visual pathways to the occipital cortex. If the macular function is normal, a delay in the p-wave suggests an optic nerve problem. The ERG measures retinal function, the b-wave originating in the Muller cells. A pattern ERG measures macular function. The EOG tests retinal pigment epithelial function. A normal Arden index is 185%.

119 **A** = False   **B** = True   **C** = True   **D** = True   **E** = True

Eyelid pathology
Solar keratosis may develop into a squamous cell carcinoma. Cellular atypia is present but not as advanced as in squamous cell carcinoma and does not invade the dermis. Basal cell carcinomata originate in the basal layer of the epidermis. They may be solid, cystic, adenoid, keratotic (with keratotic whorls) and morphoea or fibrotic types. Chalazia typically consist of granulomas with giant cells and may have fat vacuoles. The granulomatous foci may become confluent. Sarcoid granulomas are more discrete.

120   **A** = False   **B** = True   **C** = True   **D** = True   **E** = True

The **pathological changes in macular degeneration** include: thickening of Bruch's membrane; depigmentation and thinning of the retinal pigment epithelium with some pigment clumping; the deposition of PAS-positive material under the retinal pigment epithelium (drusen); distortion and loss of rods and cones. New vessels may grow through breaks in Bruch's membrane from the choroid (choroidal neovascularization). These can lead to haemorrhage and exudation beneath the RPE, in the subretinal space or within the neuroretina. Blood may even break through into the vitreous.

PAPER 3

Answers

121 **A** = True   **B** = True   **C** = False   **D** = True   **E** = True

Congenital **ptosis** is usually caused by dystrophy of the levator muscle and may be unilateral or bilateral. The dystrophic muscle both contracts and relaxes abnormally.

Disinsertion of the levator aponeurosis is the commonest acquired cause of ptosis in adults. Levator function is usually well preserved.

Myogenic		Levator disinsertion
Mild to severe	**Degree of ptosis**	Mild to severe
Reduced	**Levator function**	Normal
Absent or reduced but normal position	**Skin crease**	Elevated or absent
Lid lag	**Effect of downgaze**	Increased ptosis

Surgery for congenital myogenic ptosis requires caution because of the poor levator function. Often both sides must be operated on to achieve symmetry. For mild ptosis a Fasanella Servat or levator resection are appropriate. If levator function is severely reduced (< 5 mm) brow suspension is needed.

Aponeurotic ptosis is repaired by levator advancement or resection via an anterior or posterior approach.

122 **A** = True   **B** = True   **C** = False   **D** = False   **E** = True

Lacrimal outflow obstruction may occur at the puncta, canaliculi, sac or nasolacrimal duct.

Physiological function is tested by the Jones primary test and scintillography. Scintillography is not helpful in patients found to be blocked on syringing as an anatomical obstruction has already been identified.

With a mucocele the lacrimal sac is filled by mucoid material secondary to a nasolacrimal obstruction. This material regurgitates via the puncta with pressure over the sac. Syringing should give a 'hard stop' with regurgitation of mucus and saline on irrigation. A 'soft stop' implies obstruction of the canalicular system.

Dacryocystography is a useful test to demonstrate the site of obstruction in those patients who are found to be blocked on syringing and who do not clinically have a mucocele.

Paper 3 Answers

123 **A** = False **B** = True **C** = False **D** = True **E** = True

Axial proptosis is caused by intraconal tumours or diffuse lesions within the orbit. These include:

- **inflammatory**
    dysthyroid orbitopathy (commonest)
    orbital pseudotumour
- **vascular**
    orbital varices
    carotico-cavernous fistula
- **benign/malignant tumours**
    cavernous haemangioma
    optic nerve meningioma
    optic nerve glioma
    metastatic tumours.

Non-axial proptosis results from tumours outside the muscle cone

- **inflammatory**
    pseudotumour/myositis
- **primary tumours**
    dermoid cyst
    neurofibroma
    neurilemmoma
    haemangiopericytoma
    lymphoma
    fibrous histiocytoma
    lacrimal fossa tumour
- **invasion from adjacent structures**
    mucocele
    nasopharyngeal or sinus tumours
- **metastatic tumours.**

124 **A** = False **B** = True **C** = True **D** = True **E** = True

Periorbital oedema and ecchymosis are usually present after **blunt injury** and do not imply an orbital wall fracture. Plain X-rays of the orbits are rarely indicated. However, a fluid level in the maxillary sinus suggests orbital floor fracture with haemorrhage into the sinus.

The infra-orbital nerve runs in the floor of the orbit and is usually contused in floor fractures.

Diplopia and limitation of vertical movements result from entrapment of the inferior rectus, adjacent septae or orbital fat in the fracture site. These signs may, however, be due to oedema, haematoma or neuropathy, in which case spontaneous improvement usually occurs.

Surgical emphysema suggests a fracture resulting in communication of the orbit with one of the sinus cavities. Patients suspected of having an orbital wall fracture should be advised not to blow their nose and prophylactic oral antibiotics may be indicated. The eyes should always be carefully examined for associated injuries.

125 **A** = False   **B** = True   **C** = True   **D** = True   **E** = True

Orbital cellulitis requires urgent treatment to avoid the complications of visual loss as a result of a central retinal artery occlusion or optic nerve involvement, and even death as a result of meningitis, brain abscess and cavernous sinus thrombosis. In over 90% of cases infection spreads from the paranasal sinuses. Sphenoidal sinusitis is, however, unusual. *Haemophilus influenzae* should be considered in children under 5. *Streptococcus pneumoniae* or *Staph. aureus* are the most common organisms at other ages. CT scan may show evidence of an orbital or subperiosteal abscess requiring drainage. Sinus drainage may also be required.

126 **A** = False   **B** = True   **C** = True   **D** = True   **E** = True

Scleritis can be classified into anterior and posterior. Anterior scleritis may be diffuse or nodular, non-necrotizing or necrotizing, associated with inflammation or without (e.g. scleromalacia perforans). Scleromalacia perforans occurs in rheumatoid arthritis, is painless and causes slowly progressive scleral thinning, but seldom leads to perforation. Posterior scleritis may cause proptosis, optic disc swelling, choroidal folds, retinal exudates and exudative retinal detachments.

127 **A** = True   **B** = True   **C** = True   **D** = True   **E** = False

Vernal keratoconjunctivitis
Symblepharon is a feature of conjunctival cicatrization that does not occur in vernal keratoconjunctivitis. See answer to question 67 for more details of atopic eye disease.

128 **A** = False   **B** = True   **C** = True   **D** = False   **E** = False

Corneal dystrophies are bilateral, hereditary, progressive, primarily avascular and usually involve the central cornea. They are not associated with systemic conditions. Dystrophies are classified according to the level of cornea primarily involved.

The epithelial, subepithelial and anterior stromal dystrophies frequently cause epithelial erosions. They include:

- **epithelial and subepithelial**
    Cogan's dystrophy (map-dot fingerprint)
    Meesman's dystrophy
    recurrent erosion syndrome (this may be a dystrophy in its own right)
- **stromal**
    Reis–Buckler's (Bowman's layer)
    granular
    macular
    lattice.

The **endothelial dystrophies** may cause corneal oedema and include:

- Fuch's endothelial dystrophy
- congenital hereditary endothelial dystrophy CHED
- posterior polymorphous dystrophy.

Most of the dystrophies have autosomal dominant inheritance. However, macular dystrophy and some reported pedigrees of lattice and congenital hereditary endothelial dystrophy (CHED) are autosomal recessive.

129 **A** = True   **B** = False   **C** = False   **D** = True   **E** = True

Clinical signs in **dry eye** include:

- reduced tear meniscus height
- poor-quality tear film with excess mucus and other debris
- corneal filaments
- punctate epithelial erosions most pronounced in the interpalpebral region (Rose-Bengal may demonstrate devitalized epithelial cells better than fluorescein but often causes severe discomfort in patients with dry eye).

The normal tear film break-up time is more than 10 s (except in the presence of localized corneal irregularities). After application of topical anaesthetic the Schirmer test measures only baseline tear secretion.

In primary Sjögren's syndrome blood tests may show positive: anti Ro/ss-A, anti La/ss-B, antinuclear antibody and rheumatoid factor. Other tests may be used if specific conditions are suspected.

130 **A** = True   **B** = True   **C** = False   **D** = True   **E** = True

Peripheral corneal ulceration
In Mooren's ulcer the central edge is undermined. Scleritis secondary to one of the collagen–vascular diseases may cause corneal ulceration. Staphylococcal hypersensitivity is the commonest cause of marginal ulceration.

131 **A** = True **B** = True **C** = False **D** = False **E** = True

The following are patterns of **epithelial iron deposits**: Stoker's line with pterygium; Ferry's line with trabeculectomy; Hudson–Stahli line in old age; Fleischer's ring in keratoconus.

A Kayser–Fleischer ring is **copper** and occurs in Wilson's disease and chronic chalcosis.

Chrysiasis is due to systemic **gold** therapy (usually for rheumatoid arthritis). Gold crystals are deposited mainly in the corneal epithelium.

Argyrosis is due to **silver** that is deposited in the stroma and Descemet's membrane.

132 **A** = True **B** = True **C** = True **D** = True **E** = False

The other clinical features of **keratoconus** are Vogt's striae, fine apical white dots and Munson's sign, which is a V shape to the lower lid when the patient looks down. The main cause of a decrease in vision is irregular myopic astigmatism.

133 **A** = False **B** = True **C** = False **D** = True **E** = True

'Oil-droplet' **cataracts** are classically seen in galactosaemia where osmotic forces affect the nucleus and deep cortex. The typical cataract of myotonic dystrophy is the polychromatic 'Christmas tree' cortical cataract. Corticosteroids by any route of administration have been implicated in posterior subcapsular cataracts. The effect seems to be dose related, although individual susceptibility plays a part. Topical steroids may contribute to the posterior subcapsular cataract of uveitis.

Alkalis penetrate the anterior chamber and affect lens metabolism by raising the pH and also altering glucose and ascorbate levels.

Up to 25% of patients with atopic dermatitis develop cataracts by their third decade.

134 **A** = True **B** = False **C** = True **D** = True **E** = False

Risk factors for **failure of trabeculectomy** include:

- **strong risk factors**
    neovascular glaucoma
    previous failed filtration surgery
    uveitis (active/persistent)
    chronic conjunctival inflammation
    aphakia (intracapsular surgery)

previous topical medication (e.g. beta-blocker + pilocarpine + adrenergic agonist)
- **weaker factors**
  Afro-Caribbean race
  previous conjunctival surgery
  previous intra-ocular surgery
  young patient age (< 40) (controversial)
  previous topical medication (e.g. beta-blocker + pilocarpine)
  traumatic angle recession glaucoma.

It is important to assess the likely risk of failure so that appropriate antifibrotic measures can be used. These range from increased frequency of post-operative steroids to intraoperative application of 5-fluorouracil, mitomycin 0.02% or 0.04%, or beta-irradiation.

135   **A** = True   **B** = True   **C** = True   **D** = False   **E** = False

Aqueous flow
The intra-ocular pressure (IOP) is highest in the morning; hence, when phasing 80% will have an IOP peak between 08.00 and 12.00. Active secretion of aqueous is by non-pigmented ciliary epithelium, mainly involving a Na^+,K^+-ATPase pump to create an osmotic gradient. Carbonic anhydrase is also involved but its exact mechanism is uncertain. Twenty per cent is formed passively by ultrafiltration and diffusion. The uveoscleral route accounts for 10% of outflow. Prostaglandin analogues such as latanoprost increase this route of outflow. Pilocarpine increases flow through the trabecular route but decreases uveoscleral outflow. Ciliary body shutdown can occur with retinal detachments, ciliary body detachments, inflammation of the secretary ciliary epithelium, and with a ciliary body cleft that can occur for example with trauma.

136   **A** = False   **B** = True   **C** = True   **D** = False   **E** = True

Pigment dispersion occurs as a result of posterior bowing of the mid-peripheral iris with rubbing on the zonules. The mechanism is thought to be a reverse pupil block. The anterior chamber is deep. Pilocarpine reduces this bowing and so is an especially effective treatment. It occurs most commonly in myopic males aged 20–50 and is rare in black people. Occasionally a sudden release of pigment after exercise can cause a large spike in pressure, and so corneal oedema and haloes.

137   **A** = False   **B** = False   **C** = False   **D** = False   **E** = False

Secondary glaucoma

Ghost cell glaucoma follows vitreous haemorrhage in pseudophakes or aphakes. It involves degenerated red blood cells passing from the vitreous into the trabecular meshwork. The iridocorneal endothelium syndromes are unilateral and occur in young to middle aged women. Excessive and heavy PRP can cause choroidal effusions, which can cause secondary angle-closure glaucoma. Raised episcleral pressure occurs in Sturge–Weber syndrome and with a carotid cavernous fistula. Melanocytic glaucoma is akin to phacolytic glaucoma. Macrophages that have ingested pigment block the meshwork. In phacolytic glaucoma the macrophages have ingested lens protein.

138 **A** = False   **B** = True   **C** = True   **D** = True   **E** = False

Drug treatments of glaucoma

Beta-blockers are usually the first line of treatment for open-angle glaucoma. Betaxolol is a selective β-adrenergic blocker but all β-blockers can exacerbate asthma and so should be avoided. Pilocarpine needs to be used with caution in aphakic glaucoma as it can cause a retinal detachment. The main effects of topical treatments are

Decreased aqueous secretion	Increased outflow	
	Trabecular	Uveoscleral
β-Blockers	Pilocarpine	Brimonidine
Apraclonidine (α_2-agonist)	(parasympathetic, muscarinic agonist)	Latanoprost (prostaglandin analogue, $F_{2\alpha}$)
Brimonidine (α_2-agonist)		
Dorzolamide (carbonic anhydrase inhibitor)		

139 **A** = False   **B** = True   **C** = True   **D** = False   **E** = True

On ultrasound, a **uveal melanoma** has low internal reflectivity, reflecting its homogeneous consistency. A haemangioma by contrast has high internal reflectivity. Choroidal excavation on ultrasound is a typical feature of a melanoma. It is an artefact caused by the way that sound waves travel through the tumour and is not reflected by the pathological findings. Internal vascularity may best be seen by small movements in the internal signal from the lesion on A-scan. The shape of the lesion may be characteristic, for example 'collar stud' tumours. A mildly elevated lobulated shape is more characteristic of a metastasis. Extra-scleral extension may be found.

140 **A** = False   **B** = False   **C** = False   **D** = True   **E** = True

Endophthalmitis following cataract surgery most commonly occurs between 48 and 72 hours after surgery. The most common pathogen is *Staph. epidermidis*. Late-onset endophthalmitis, which may run a more indolent course and be treated as recurrent iritis, is often caused by *Propionibacterium acnes*. Acute endophthalmitis should be managed with a vitreous biopsy and injection of intravitreal antibiotics. The current recommendations are for vancomycin and amikacin. Gentamicin should be avoided as it is highly retinotoxic on intracameral use. Primary or early vitrectomy has been recommended in severe cases. Infections following trabeculectomy are more common if an antimetabolite has been used (up to 4% risk per year after surgery with mitomycin C). With treated *Staph. epidermidis* endophthalmitis 60% should regain some useful vision. With streptococci the prognosis is very poor.

141   A = True   B = True   C = True   D = True   E = False

In **Fuch's heterochromic cyclitis** signs include: diffuse stellate KPs; heterochromia, iris nodules; iris transillumination; no posterior synechiae; abnormal vessels in the angle that may bleed on entering the eye in surgery (Amsler's sign); vitreous cells. Visual loss is due to cataract and glaucoma but vitreous opacities can also be a problem. Cystoid macular oedema is rare.

142   A = True   B = True   C = True   D = True   E = False

In non-accidental injury **retinal haemorrhages** may occur, especially around the disc and in the peripheral retina. There is a strong correlation with these and the presence of intracranial bleeds.

143   A = True   B = True   C = True   D = False   E = True

Choroidal neovascularization (CNV) can occur in any condition that affects the integrity of the choriocapillaris–Bruch's–retinal pigment epithelium–outer retinal complex. Specific causes include:

- **idiopathic**
- **inflammatory**, punctate inner choroidopathy (PIC), multifocal choroiditis (MIC), *Toxoplasma* retinochoroiditis
- **traumatic**, choroidal rupture
- **degenerative**, age-related macular degeneration, myopia, angioid streaks, optic nerve drusen
- **neoplastic**, choroidal naevi and melanomas
- **iatrogenic**, retinal photocoagulation.

144 **A** = True **B** = True **C** = True **D** = True **E** = True

Central serous chorioretinopathy (CSCR) is more common in the third to fourth decade in 'type A' men. It causes distortion of central vision, a central or paracentral scotoma, micropsia, and may be improved by a +1-dioptre lens. It can occur in association with an optic disc pit. Fluorescein angiography may reveal one leaking point. This can be treated with focal laser if appropriate, although a CSCR will usually settle with no treatment. ICG shows a much more widespread disease, often affecting both eyes.

145 **A** = True **B** = True **C** = True **D** = True **E** = True

Diabetic retinopathy
These figures are influenced in the individual patient by other factors such as the control of blood sugar levels, hypertension, carotid vascular disease and pregnancy.

146 **A** = True **B** = True **C** = False **D** = True **E** = True

Sickle cell trait is relatively common in the black population. Retinopathy is most common in SC disease, probably because the anaemia is not so severe and so blood viscosity higher.

147 **A** = True **B** = True **C** = True **D** = True **E** = True

Conditions with **deafness and retinitis pigmentosa** include:

- Usher's syndrome
- Alstrom's syndrome
- Bardet–Biedl syndrome
- Refsum's disease
- retinal–renal disease
- Leber's congenital amaurosis
- mitochondrial myopathies
- congenital rubella
- mucopolysaccharidoses.

148 **A** = True **B** = True **C** = True **D** = False **E** = True

Macular exudate may accumulate with

- widespread or diffuse retinal vascular disease, as occurs with, for example, diabetes mellitus and severe hypertension

- focal central vascular abnormalities, e.g. a branch retinal vein occlusion, choroidal neovascularization, retinal telangiectasia, macroaneurysm
- a leak from a peripheral vascular abnormality, e.g. from a capillary haemangioma in von Hippel–Lindau disease or Coat's disease.

149 **A** = True   **B** = True   **C** = True   **D** = False   **E** = True

The diagnosis of an ischaemic **CRVO** is mainly clinical: poor visual acuity (usually count fingers or worse), a relative afferent pupil defect, extensive haemorrhages and cotton wool spots. Electroretinography can also be helpful, especially if serial measurements are performed. A fundus fluorescein angiogram may help but the picture is often obscured by haemorrhage. An area of ten disc diameters of non-perfusion is diagnostic of ischaemia. About 50% are non-ischaemic on presentation, although about 12% may subsequently convert to the ischaemic type. This is more common over 65 years of age. In younger patients there is a lower incidence of ischaemia and the visual prognosis is better. Aspirin should be avoided at the acute stage as it can make the haemorrhage worse, but should be considered later for prophylaxis.

150 **A** = True   **B** = False   **C** = False   **D** = False   **E** = False

The first phase of a **fluorescein angiogram** is choroidal, followed by arterial, capillary and venous. It takes 6–8 s for dye to reach the retinal circulation (although this time may be prolonged in severe vascular disease). Dye reaches the choroidal circulation 1 s earlier. It is important that photographs are taken from 5 s after injection so that the early phases are seen. The disc stains because of leakage of dye from the peripapillary choroidal plexus. If an anaphylactic reaction occurs the dose of adrenaline required is 0.5 ml of 1:1000 given intramuscularly. The dose in the question is that used for cardiac resuscitation and is given intravenously.

151 **A** = True   **B** = True   **C** = True   **D** = True   **E** = False

Retinal vasculitis involves inflammation of the vessels, most commonly the veins. Clinically the vessels may be sheathed and there may be leakage. This leakage can be seen more easily with fluorescein angiography. The area involved may become ischaemic and so neovascularization may be found. The underlying pathology of multiple sclerosis is a periphlebitis. Vascular sheathing is seen in the peripheral retina. In sarcoidosis, venous sheathing with skip lesions is classically seen.

152 **A** = True **B** = True **C** = True **D** = False **E** = False

Carriers of genetic disease
To offer genetic counselling a clear family history is required and family members need to be screened. Electrodiagnostic tests may be appropriate even with a normal fundal appearance. This is the case in Best's disease, in which carriers often have an abnormal EOG. Peripheral RPE atrophy may occur in carriers of choroideraemia and in X-linked ocular albinism where iris transillumination may also be seen.

153 **A** = True **B** = False **C** = False **D** = True **E** = True

Macular holes are commonest in the sixth to eighth decades. The underlying pathology is thought to be tangential vitreomacular traction. Gass classified macular holes into four main stages:

- **stage 1**, impending hole
    - **1a**, yellow dot at fovea
    - **1b**, yellow ring at fovea
- **stage 2**, central, full-thickness hole < 400 μm diameter
- **stage 3**, central, full-thickness hole > 400 μm diameter
- **stage 4**, as stage 3 plus posterior vitreous detachment.

Macular holes become bilateral with time in about 25–30% of cases. Vitrectomy is not indicated for stage 1 holes because spontaneous resolution commonly occurs. Vitrectomy with peeling of any premacular membranes and post-operative gas tamponade may improve visual acuity in stage 2, 3 and 4 holes.

154 **A** = True **B** = True **C** = True **D** = True **E** = True

Retinal lesions associated with **increased risk of rhegmatogenous detachment** include:

- lattice degeneration
- vitreoretinal tufts
- white without pressure
- diffuse chorioretinal atrophy.

Infections that can predispose to retinal detachment include
- CMV retinitis (leads to RD in 20%)
- AIDS (5% risk)
- acute retinal necrosis.

Inherited syndromes with increased risk of retinal detachment are

- Jansen's
- Stickler's
- Marfan's
- Ehlers–Danlos
- Goldman–Favre
- homocystinuria.

Other factors that increase the risk of retinal detachment are

- myopes (42% of all RDs)
- post-cataract surgery (1.4% risk in uncomplicated ECCE)
- YAG laser capsulotomy (2.3% risk)
- blunt trauma especially with hyphaema
- RD in fellow eye (very important).

155 A = False   B = False   C = True   D = True   E = False

The main differential of a **retinoschisis** is of a longstanding rhegmatogenous retinal detachment. The following features help make the distinction. Retinoschisis is usually inferior temporal and often bilateral. A pigmented demarcation line suggests a longstanding rhegmatogenous retinal detachment, not retinoschisis. Fine white dots on the inner leaf are common. If the retinoschisis extends posterior to the equator there will be an absolute visual field defect. Patients are more likely to be hypermetropic, unlike those with retinal detachment.

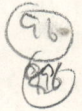

156 A = False   B = True   C = False   D = False   E = True

Assessment of a **squint** should include cycloplegic refraction (in children) and ocular examination including fundoscopy. An esotropia should be given a full hypermetropic correction and an exotropia a full myopic correction. If amblyopia is present this should be treated before squint surgery. Congenital esotropias have a poor prognosis for binocular single vision even with early treatment.

A near esotropia can be caused by

- accommodative esotropia with convergence excess (high AC/A ratio)
- non-accommodative convergence excess (normal AC/A ratio)
- undercorrected hypermetropia.

157 A = True   B = False   C = False   D = True   E = True

Exotropias are often intermittent and so not usually associated with amblyopia. A 'V' pattern is more common with a distance exotropia.

Exotropias can be classified as

- primary
- consecutive (following an esotropia, e.g. after surgery or spontaneously)
- secondary (following severe visual loss).

158 **A** = True **B** = True **C** = True **D** = False **E** = True

For corneas to be stored in organ culture for up to 28 days the following medical contraindications apply:

- **infections**
    HIV/AIDS and donors in high-risk groups
    active viral hepatitis B or C
    viral seropositivity for HIV, HbsAg, HCV
    Creutzfeldt–Jakob disease
    recipients of human pituitary growth hormone
    rabies
    congenital rubella
    tuberculosis
    Reye's syndrome
- **CNS disorders of unknown aetiology**
- **death from unknown cause** (unless a post-mortem is to be performed)
- **malignancies**
    leukaemia, lymphoma, myeloma
- **intrinsic eye disease**
    ocular inflammation
    congenital or acquired ocular disorders that would preclude successful graft outcome
    retinoblastoma
    malignant tumours of the anterior segment
    previous intra-ocular surgery.

For corneas to be stored shorter term at 4°C septicaemia is also a contraindication to donation.

159 **A** = False **B** = True **C** = False **D** = True **E** = False

The mean **refractive error** in the newborn is +2 dioptres with a normal distribution. Emmetropia gradually develops with little change in refraction after the age of 13. Six per cent of 1-year-olds have a significant refractive error and most of these are hyperopic. Hyperopia may be overestimated in the infant eye as the retinoscopy reflex is thought to arise anterior to the retina at the internal limiting membrane and the error created by this is magnified if the eye is smaller. Astigmatism is common in infancy and is usually against the rule. By the age of 5 the prevalence of astigmatism is similar to that in adults. Cyclopentolate 0.5% should be used for cycloplegia before the age of 3 months and 1% thereafter. Atropine 1% ointment given for the 3 days before retinoscopy may be needed in heavily pigmented eyes.

160 **A** = False **B** = False **C** = True **D** = True **E** = True

Recessive **RP** results in the most severe visual loss, with night blindness in childhood, extensive field loss by teens, central visual loss by the twenties and central vision less than counting fingers by the fourth decade. X-linked RP is very variable, and autosomal dominant RP rarely causes problems until later life. EOG is difficult to perform in young children, and unlike ERG shows only minimal changes early in the disease. ERG provides objective evidence of severity of retinal impairment. Typical changes are: reduction in both rod and cone responses, reduction in both a- and b-waves and prolongation of b-waves.

Other clinical features such as deafness (e.g. Usher's syndrome) and neurological impairment (e.g. Friedreich's ataxia) should be sought and tested for if necessary.

In Refsum's disease the neurological sequelae may be reduced by avoidance of dietary phytanic acid, whereas in abetalipoproteinaemia vitamin A and E supplements may prevent both retinal and neurological complications.

Complications of RP include cystoid macular oedema (CMO) and posterior subcapsular cataracts. The CMO may respond to acetazolamide treatment.

161 **A** = True **B** = True **C** = False **D** = True **E** = True

Retinopathy of prematurity
Between 30% and 60% of babies < 1500 g develop some degree of retinopathy, with severe disease virtually limited to babies < 1500 g and < 31 weeks gestational age.

Stage 1 disease is the development of a demarcation line between vascularized and non-vascularized retina. This usually develops in the temporal retina as the nasal retina is already vascularized, except in the very premature. In **stage 2** this line becomes a ridge and in **stage 3** extra-retinal fibrovascular proliferation occurs. **Plus disease** is the presence of iris vessel engorgement, vitreous haze and dilated retinal vessels. **Threshold disease** is defined as stage 3 ROP involving five or more contiguous, or eight or more interrupted clock hours in the presence of 'plus' disease. Of 6600 babies born < 1500 g in the UK each year, 80% (5280) survive and 8–10% (450) develop stage 3 ROP.

Treatment involves laser or cryotherapy to the non-vascularized area of retina. This reduces the incidence of blindness by 50%.

162 **A** = True **B** = False **C** = True **D** = False **E** = False

In a large series of **children with proptosis**, 16% were tumours, the rest being developmental abnormalities such as craniosynostosis, inflammatory, metabolic such as hyperthyroidism and generalized disease such as histiocytosis X and fibrous dysplasia.

Acute or rapidly progressive proptosis is seen in orbital cellulitis. However, rhabdomyosarcoma or metastatic disease should be suspected. Unilateral proptosis is more likely to be due to an orbital mass, whereas bilateral proptosis is more likely to be developmental. CT scanning is useful for bone imaging and is often easier to perform in children.

Café-au-lait spots are a feature of neurofibromatosis.

163 **A** = True **B** = True **C** = True **D** = False **E** = False

Jaw claudication is pathognomonic for **temporal arteritis** but needs to be distinguished from tempero-mandibular joint pain. Tongue infarction can occur, as can scalp necrosis over occluded temporal arteries. Other arteries can also be affected including coronary arteries, causing angina; leg arteries, causing claudication; and mesenteric vessels, causing abdominal pain. Other ocular features of temporal arteritis are: central retinal artery occlusion, cotton wool spots, amaurosis fugax, cortical blindness and ocular motor palsies. Nail-bed splinter haemorrhages suggest subacute bacterial endocarditis, which can also cause a high ESR. Erythema nodosa occur with sarcoidosis, which could affect the optic nerve.

164 **A** = True **B** = True **C** = True **D** = True **E** = False

There is asymmetry of the **OKN** response with a parietal lobe lesion and with congenital esotropia. In occipital lesions the OKN response is usually symmetrical. In convergence retraction nystagmus (e.g. in dorsal midbrain syndrome) downward rotation of the OKN drum causes spasmodic convergence.

165 **A** = True **B** = True **C** = True **D** = False **E** = True

Myasthenia gravis
A tensilon test is useful, but, especially in disease localized to the eye, it may be negative. Acetylcholine receptor antibodies may be detected in the serum. A good test is single-fibre EMG, which shows characteristic changes. The CSF is normal. A similar pattern to myasthenia can occur with the Miller–Fisher variant of the Guillain–Barré syndrome. In this condition the CSF is abnormal.

166 **A** = True **B** = False **C** = False **D** = True **E** = True

Carotico-cavernous fistulae may be high or slow flow (direct or indirect). High-flow fistulae are due to a direct communication between the internal carotid artery and the cavernous sinus and may occur after trauma. Slow-flow fistulae are more common and often occur as a result of shunt vessels between dural vessels of the carotid artery and the cavernous sinus, and usually occur spontaneously. Most slow-flow fistulae will settle without intervention. Management is aimed at controlling the complications, in particular open-angle glaucoma. Other causes of visual loss are corneal exposure caused by proptosis, venous stasis retinopathy, optic neuropathy and ophthalmoplegia. Rarely, angle-closure glaucoma can occur as a result of choroidal detachments.

167 **A** = True **B** = True **C** = True **D** = False **E** = True

Optic disc drusen are nearly always bilateral and are found in up to 1% of the white population, but very rarely in black or coloured people. Autosomal dominant inheritance with incomplete penetrance may be found. Ocular associations include some forms of retinitis pigmentosa and angioid streaks. Visual field loss may be present.

Buried drusen may be confused with papilloedema. However, superficial drusen have a characteristic appearance. Superficial drusen display autofluorescence with cobalt blue light, whereas orbital CT scanning or B-scan ultrasound demonstrate the presence of buried drusen.

Visual loss may occur as a result of vascular occlusions, subretinal neovascularization, anterior ischaemic optic neuropathy or progressive optic neuropathy.

168 **A** = True **B** = True **C** = True **D** = True **E** = True

Herpes zoster ophthalmicus can affect all aspects of ocular function, as well as causing neurological complications. A person who has not previously had chickenpox can catch it from a patient with shingles. This can be a problem for pregnant women in the first and second trimesters especially.

169 **A** = True **B** = False **C** = True **D** = True **E** = False

NF2 has autosomal dominant inheritance with incomplete penetrance. The gene defect is located on chromosome 22. Diagnostic criteria are

- either
    bilateral acoustic nerve masses

- or
    first-degree relative with NF2
- and
    unilateral acoustic nerve mass
- or at least two of
    meningioma
    Schwannoma
    glioma
    neurofibroma
    posterior subcapsular cataract.

170 **A** = True   **B** = False   **C** = False   **D** = True   **E** = True

Essential blepharospasm is nearly always bilateral and causes mild twitches of the eyelids, which progress to marked orbicularis spasm. Functional blindness may occur as a result of the prolonged eye closure. The differential diagnosis includes eyelid closure caused by dry eye and other ocular surface disorders, and hemifacial spasm (see below). Treatment is largely medical by injection of botulinum toxin to the orbcularis muscle. This needs to be repeated at 3- to 4-monthly intervals. Unresponsive cases may require surgical myectomy of the orbicularis muscle or facial nerve stripping.

Essential blepharospasm		Hemifacial spasm
F > M	**Sex**	M > F
> 50	**Age**	> 50
Bilateral	**Laterality**	Unilateral (commonly left-sided)
No	**Present in sleep**	Yes
Central dystonia	**Pathogenesis**	Facial nerve root compression

171 **A** = False   **B** = True   **C** = False   **D** = True   **E** = True

An **afferent pupil defect** (APD) is caused by a lesion in the afferent pathway from the retina to the Edinger–Westphal nucleus in the midbrain. The degree of APD corresponds to the extent of ganglion cell loss. These fibres decussate at the chiasm and again in the midbrain, and lesions anterior to the chiasm that are either unilateral or assymmetric result in a **'relative' afferent pupil defect** (i.e. an APD of one side relative to the other).

Causes of RAPD include asymmetric

- **retinal pathology**
    vascular occlusions
    large retinal scars

extensive maculopathy
retinal detachment
- **optic nerve**
  glaucoma
  ischaemic optic neuropathy
  optic neuritis
  optic nerve tumours or compression
- **anterior chiasmal lesions**
  RAPD is not caused by
- refractive errors
- media opacities
- functional visual loss
- cortical lesions.

172 **A** = False **B** = True **C** = False **D** = True **E** = True

Ocular conditions more common in pregnancy
Inflammatory and autoimmune conditions frequently improve markedly during pregnancy but may flare up during the post-partum period. Exudative retinal detachments may occur during pregnancy.

173 **A** = True **B** = True **C** = False **D** = True **E** = True

Congenital nystagmus may be classified as sensory or motor. Pathology affecting image formation at the macula, or of the afferent visual pathways, may cause **sensory nystagmus**. The severity of nystagmus often reflects the degree of visual impairment and when poor vision is present from birth nystagmus appears in the first few months of life.

Motor nystagmus results from a defect in central motor control or the efferent mechanisms and usually appears soon after birth. No ocular abnormalities are associated. Clinically the movement is of the 'jerk' type. Different directions of gaze often affect the degree of nystagmus and a 'null position' of minimal nystagmus may be found. This null position may lead to an abnormal head posture. Convergence may damp nystagmus with resultant improvement in visual acuity for near.

Spasmus nutans consists of nystagmus, involuntary head movements and an abnormal head posture. It usually resolves spontaneously by 3 years of age, but occasionally it can be associated with a chiasmal glioma. It therefore requires investigation.

174 **A** = False   **B** = True   **C** = False   **D** = False   **E** = True

Retinal laser treatment
Retinal burns of 100 μm and from 200 to 500 μm in the periphery are generally used. The spot diameter affects the area of retina treated and the power required to create a burn. Larger spot sizes require higher laser power as the energy is spread over a larger area. Doubling the spot diameter results in a fourfold increase in the area treated, so knowledge of the magnifying power of the lens used is essential. In general, all lenses used increase the retinal spot size relative to the setting on the laser. The Goldman three-mirror lens has the least effect.

Lens	**Magnification factor on burn diameter**
Rodenstock Panfundoscope	2.0
Volk Quadraspheric	1.92
Mainster Ultrafield	1.89
Mainster wide field lens	1.47
Goldman standard three-mirror lens	1.08

175 **A** = False   **B** = False   **C** = False   **D** = True   **E** = True

For a standard **car licence** the driver has to be able to read a clean number plate with letters 3.5 inches high at 25 yards in bright daylight with glasses, if worn. The visual fields should be 120° horizontally and 20° above and below the horizontal meridian using a 3-mm white test object at 1/3 m (III 4e on Goldman). Colour vision defects are not a bar to driving.

176 **A** = False   **B** = False   **C** = True   **D** = True   **E** = True

Laser settings
In general the lowest laser power or energy to achieve the required effect should be used.
   YAG capsulotomy should be started with an energy setting of 0.5–1 mJ and the setting increased until adequate photodisruption of the posterior capsule occurs. Using a defocus setting reduces the likelihood of pitting or cracking the implant.
   YAG iridotomy is best achieved with a small number of shots. Using several pulses per burst aimed at the base of a peripheral iris crypt in the superior iris may create an iridotomy with only one or two shots.
   With the **argon laser,** reducing the spot size concentrates the energy on to a smaller area so that the power may need to be reduced to avoid excessive reaction.
Argon PRP is often best performed at two sittings a few weeks apart. Where there is imminent risk of vitreous haemorrhage treat the lower retina first as the view of this area may be obscured when the patient is next seen.

Paper 3 Answers

Trabeculoplasty needs a small spot size of 50 μm and high power of 500 mW or more. For macular grid laser a medium to small spot size of 100 μm and a time of 0.1 s are appropriate. Argon green should be used to avoid excessive absorption by the xanthophil pigment in the inner retinal layers, with just enough power to create faint blanching.

177 **A** = True   **B** = True   **C** = True   **D** = True   **E** = True

Associations of myopia
Neonatal visual deprivation blocks the process of emmetropization and can lead to myopia. Other associations are

- **ocular**
    retinopathy of prematurity
    choroideraemia
    retinitis pigmentosa
    ectopia lentis
- **systemic**
    Marfan's syndrome
    Weill–Marchesani
    homocystinuria
    Ehlers–Danlos
    Pierre Robin
    Down's syndrome.

178 **A** = True   **B** = False   **C** = False   **D** = False   **E** = True

Inheritance
Stargardt's and Usher's are autosomal recessive, and juvenile retinoschisis is X-linked recessive.

179 **A** = True   **B** = True   **C** = False   **D** = True   **E** = True

Tumours occurring at the limbus may be benign, precancerous or malignant. Choristomas may also be found. These are the continued growth of normal tissue that has been displaced as a result of a developmental error. Examples are dermoid tumours and dermolipomas that can occur at the limbus. Other benign lesions are papilloma and keratotic plaques and, rarely, neurofibroma, haemangiomata, fibroxanthomata and neurolemmomata. Carcinoma *in situ* can occur as well as squamous cell carcinoma.

180 **A** = True   **B** = True   **C** = True   **D** = True   **E** = False

Pigmented lesions
Oculodermal melanocytosis (naevus of Ota) is unilateral with pigmentation of the skin, eyelids, episclera, sclera and uvea. Malignant change is rare but has been reported. Conjunctival naevi occur most commonly at the limbus and the caruncle. They may be junctional or compound. Primary acquired melanosis can have no atypical cells and clinically be just an area of pigmentation, or it can have marked atypia and grow more rapidly and so can be precancerous. Episcleral melanosis is congenital and typically has a slate-blue colour. The conjunctiva can be moved over the area. Malignant change would be very rare indeed.